CONTENTS

⩗ W9-BVR-741

Preface, v

Introduction, 1

1. What Are Migraines?, 13

2. Bioidentical Remedies, 21

- Riboflavin, 21
- Coenzyme Q_{10}, 30
- Magnesium, 35
- Melatonin, 43
- 5-Hydroxytryptamine (5-HTP), 46
- Niacin, 53
- Vitamin D, 59

3. Herbal Remedies, 67

- Feverfew, 67
- White Willow, 74
- Butterbur, 78
- Ginger, 83
- Ginkgo Biloba, 87
- Gamma Linoleic Acid (GLA), 89

4. Mind and Body Remedies, 93

- Biofeedback, 93
- Acupuncture, 101

5. Preventing Migraines in Children and Adolescents, 107

6. Natural Remedies for Acute Migraines, 117

Conclusion, 130

References, 137

About the Author, 148

Index, 149

PREFACE

My medical odyssey has included general medicine, pain research, pharmacology, psychiatry, and psychopharmacology. Yet it was my personal experience with migraine headaches that led me to write this book, which contains information I've collected over the last fifteen years.

My desire to release this information arose when my occasional severe migraines disappeared in 1995. At the time, I had begun to use magnesium in the treatment of another serious medical problem. I knew there had to be a connection. Amazingly, I have not experienced a migraine since then. Once in a while, however, I am reminded that the condition lurks inside me. For example, I sometimes develop visual aura when I glance at the summer sunlight by the pool where I swim. If I eat too much dark chocolate, migraine pain threatens to return, but fades quickly.

I have personally tried many of the natural remedies discussed in this book, obtaining benefits from some but not others. I do not expect every therapy to work for me or anyone else. One of the cardinal aspects of migraines, and of many other medical conditions, is that different treatments work for different people. Migraine sufferers have to try a variety of

options carefully and thoughtfully, one by one, allow-
ing enough time for a therapy to work.

Natural remedies can provide people with quick
improvement, but sometimes positive results take
weeks or months. More often than not, it requires
three to six months to see the full benefits of a natural
therapy. In one study of coenzyme Q_{10}, the average
frequency of subjects' migraines decreased by only 13
percent after one month of treatment. By the end of
the third month, however, the frequency of migraine
headaches dropped by 55 percent on average. For
some subjects, the rate fell far more. These are excellent results, equaling or surpassing those of many
migraine drugs. When it comes to natural remedies,
patience is indeed a virtue.

Why does it take so long to see results? It is
because, unlike drugs, natural therapies have to pene-
trate the body's fifty trillion cells and gradually build
up tissue levels. This takes time. Yet, some people
show improvements within days or weeks of starting
a natural therapy. There is no rule of thumb.

My goal in writing this book is to provide you
with substantial, scientifically validated information
that has been peer reviewed and published in medical
journals. These high-quality medical facts conform to
the current definition of "evidence-based medicine"
and can make it easy for you to choose and use one or
more natural remedies for your migraines. Armed
with this information, you can prevent your migraines
before they start, or stop them once they have started.

It may surprise you to learn that many natural
migraine remedies are as effective as pharmaceuticals.

Plus, they do not require a prescription, can be obtained at health food stores, and do not produce the side effects that come with taking migraine drugs.

In the United States alone, 49 percent of people use alternative medicine. Clearly, alternative methods of therapy are widely accepted. You would think that mainstream medicine would be equally open to the use of treatments that are natural to the body, proven by scientific research, and much safer and less expensive than prescription drugs. But the reality is that few doctors know about these natural solutions, and fewer still recommend them to their patients.

My goal in writing this book is to help you, the consumer, find safe, effective ways to treat your migraines, and to provide high-quality, medically valid information that may open doctors' eyes to safer ways to treat this vicious condition. We've got nothing to lose but our migraines.

Jay S. Cohen, MD

INTRODUCTION

Why don't doctors prescribe natural remedies for migraine headaches? After all, safety is the first concern of people when they are prescribed a medication. Safety should also be the first concern of their doctors, yet often it is not. Doctors may protest that safety is their first concern, but their actions, unfortunately, say otherwise.

Propranolol is a frequently prescribed medication for preventing migraines. Yet propranolol can cause your gums to recede enough to alarm your dentist. It can reduce your ability to exercise by half. A brief list of the hundreds of adverse effects that can occur with propranolol include vertigo, fatigue, headache, mental depression, peripheral nerve abnormality, anxiety, impaired concentration, nightmares, gastritis, hair loss, nausea, sweating, sexual dysfunction, liver irritation, joint pain, muscle cramps, burning eyes, facial swelling, and cardiac arrhythmia.[1]

In contrast, riboflavin is a natural substance made in small amounts by your own body. Therefore, supplemental riboflavin is a bioidentical remedy, which means your body does not react to it as a foreign substance. As such, its side effects are rare. Riboflavin and propranolol are equally effective in preventing migraines. If given a choice, which treatment would you try first to prevent your migraines? The riboflavin, of course. Yet, which would your doctor choose first? Likely, the propranolol.

MORE THAN AN INFORMATION GAP

You might think that doctors stick with the medication-first approach because they do not possess enough information about natural remedies. Yet, how can this be, when medical journals first reported the benefits of magnesium in 1933, of niacin in 1944, and of riboflavin in 1946? In fact, there is plenty of evidence, including multiple studies in medical journals, of the effectiveness of many natural therapies. For half a century, ample proof has been available regarding the benefits of magnesium or niacin given intravenously for acute migraines, yet emergency doctors persist in using injectable drugs that have dangerous, sometimes lethal, side effects.

Natural Remedies for Migraines and the Years Medical Journals First Reported Their Benefits

Magnesium: 1933	Vitamin D: 1994
Niacin: 1944	Gamma linolenic acid: 1997
Riboflavin: 1946	Butterbur: 2000
Biofeedback: 1972	Coenzyme Q10: 2002
5-HTP: 1973	Melatonin: 2004
Feverfew: 1985	White willow: 2006
Ginger: 1990	Alpha lipoic acid: 2007
Acupuncture: 1992	Ginkgo biloba: 2009

A basic principle of optimal medical care is to use the safest remedies first for people with health problems. So why don't doctors embrace these effective natural treatments for their migraine patients? Why not try these safer approaches first and then go to a prescription drug if necessary?

WHAT IS RELIABLE EVIDENCE?

Most doctors are good people who want to help their patients. The problem is not doctors' intentions, but the sources of information and other influences from which doctors make treatment decisions. In recent years, mainstream medicine has adopted a new standard of medical care known as evidence-based medicine. This standard makes sense and is long overdue, as studies of doctors' methods have shown that their decision-making is often unscientific. Physicians are now encouraged to make treatment choices based on reliable, evidence-based information.

Yet, what information do doctors accept as evidence-based? If you were to ask them what "evidence-based medicine" means, many would say it means using only the findings of big drug company-run studies. Unfortunately, throughout their training, future physicians are taught that big studies are the sole source of information worth considering. This viewpoint is flawed. While these large reports can produce good data, they often have many flaws and can mislead the medical profession and the public. The following list details the ways in which major drug company studies may be unreliable.

- **Biased Comparisons.** Drug companies compare their new drugs to older, less effective drugs. This makes their products appear better than they actually are.

- **Favorably Designed Studies.** Drug companies can design their studies to obtain better outcomes. They can also avoid doing important research that might reveal unfavorable results or serious risks of a drug. Studies conducted by the manufacturer of a drug being researched frequently yield more favorable results than do independent studies.

- **Manipulating Measurements of Effectiveness.** Drug companies can employ several measures of effectiveness, and then pick and choose the most favorable ones while suppressing those that are unfavorable. The new drug is then promoted with a misleadingly positive profile.

- **Non-Representative Subjects.** Drug studies are sometimes conducted with young, healthy subjects rather than older subjects, even if the new drug will be used primarily by older patients. Young subjects usually report better rates of improvement and fewer side effects. This provides impressive yet inaccurate data about the benefits of the drug.

- **Publication of Only Favorable Studies.** Drug companies can pick and choose among multiple studies, publishing only the most favorable ones.

- **Stacking Data.** A limited amount of favorable data about a drug can be amplified by repackaging the information into different articles by different authors in different journals, creating the impression that the favorable data are considerable when, in fact, the results are limited.

- **Suppression of Vital Information.** If a study's results aren't to a drug company's liking, that company can suppress the data or impede publication of the report. It can also keep a study from public awareness by declaring it "proprietary information." Some researchers determined to publish important side-effect warnings have even been threatened with lawsuits or the loss of their jobs.

Doctors are generally unaware of these problems. Prospective physicians are trained to copy the methods of their teachers. They are not educated to ask questions or seek better ideas. Furthermore, medical schools have become increasingly reliant on research funding from drug companies, and medical school teachers, many of whom are recipients of drug company handouts, often share their drug-first view of medical therapy with their students.

In light of these facts, it has been easy to convince doctors that only studies sponsored by drug companies are worth believing. The irony, however, is that pharmaceutical companies are forced by the US Food and Drug Administration (FDA) to conduct large studies that involve thousands of patients because their drugs run a high risk of being toxic. In contrast, natural therapies do not require large studies because of their high degree of safety. Yet, the pharmaceutical industry has been able to turn this reality on its head, convincing doctors that reports of natural remedies are not large enough to be credible. The result of unrelenting propaganda of this nature is that many doctors have closed their minds to important information about natural remedies.

A woman recently told me, "When I told my doctor that magnesium had greatly reduced my migraines, my doctor said, 'That's nice,' and then changed the subject. I had hoped he would be interested enough to tell his other migraine patients, but he wasn't interested."

I have heard stories like this from dozens of patients. Doctors have been trained to be skeptical about any individual reports because they do not consider them reliable, or, in other words, evidence-based. Indeed, physicians have learned to dismiss individual reports and sneer at any data termed "anecdotal." This narrow-mindedness often includes cases mentioned in medical journals, even though these articles have been peer reviewed, which means they have been read and approved by other doctors before being accepted for publication.

Consider this: Most people with long histories of migraines have usually tried every substance under the sun, including prescription pharmaceuticals, over-the-counter drugs, and dietary supplements, seeking relief. If nothing has worked, it is obvious that these people are not susceptible to the placebo effect that can occur as a result of trying a new potential remedy. When such a person tries a new therapy and it works, I consider this response to be highly significant, provided the benefits last at least six months. And you can bet I mention this treatment to other migraine sufferers.

It is odd that doctors have been trained to disdain individual reports. A person's own experience can be as valuable, or even more valuable, than the results of elaborate studies. So, the next time your doctor dismisses your experience with a natural remedy, remind him that the FDA places a high value on the anecdotal case stories it receives. When it comes to the public's safety, the FDA will ban a drug if it receives enough reports of serious harm or death from the substance, no matter if the drug manufacturer has conducted fifty major studies attesting to the safety of the pharmaceutical. If the FDA puts such weight on individual experiences, why don't doctors?

EVIDENCE-BASED MEDICINE: WHAT IT IS AND WHAT IT IS NOT

Believing solely in evidence provided by large corporate-sponsored studies can be counterproductive and harmful to patients. If doctors trust only drug company-generated reports, their treatment decisions will be drugs first, second, and third. I am not against medications, which help millions of people, but I am against a medication-first mentality when there are other, safer, evidence-based options.

Maybe doctors should be reminded what the term evidence-based medicine actually means. Here is an appropriate definition written by experts in a book titled *Evidence-Based Medicine: What It Is and What It Isn't*:

The practice of evidence-based medicine means integrating individual clinical expertise with the best available external clinical evidence from sys-

tematic research. . . . Good doctors use both individual clinical expertise and the best available
external evidence, and neither alone is enough. . . .
Evidence-based medicine is not restricted to randomized trials and meta-analyses.[2]

What this means, in effect, is that clinical experience, which refers to experience treating individuals,
is as important as big studies. And this definition does
not stand alone. Many other experts have echoed the
idea that big drug-company studies are not the only
valid source of information. Individual experiences
count. Small studies count. Open label studies, in
which doctors and patients know what the treatment
is, count. Retrospective analyses count. Epidemiologi-
cal studies count. Each of these sources is important.
Your experiences count!

Recently, a patient of mine, a very bright doctor of
psychology, showed her medical doctor a study
involving a natural remedy for pain. The results of the
study were excellent, but her physician rejected the
results because the study was "too small." The study
involved 450 subjects. It was not a small study for a
natural remedy. But this doctor's mind was made up,
having bought in long ago to the drug-company line
that says only huge studies count. That's what he was
taught, and that's what he wanted to believe. In doing
so, he had closed the door on anything other than prescription pharmaceuticals—despite scientifically valid
evidence to the contrary.

When physicians dismiss studies because they are
"too small," or personal experiences because they are
"anecdotal," they violate the basic tenets of evidence-

What Evidence-Based Medicine Really Means

"Evidence-based medicine is the integration of best research evidence with clinical expertise and patient values."
—*Evidence-Based Medicine: How to Practice and Teach EBM*[3]

"Evidence-based medicine has been defined as 'the integration of the best research evidence with clinical expertise and patient values.' Unfortunately, it is considered by many [doctors] to be synonymous with reviews and guidelines produced in 'ivory towers' with questionable local applicability and relevance to the personal circumstances of many patients."
—*Emergency Medicine Australasia*[4]

"The practice of medicine is in effect the conducting of clinical research. . . . Every practicing physician conducts clinical trials daily as he is seeing patients. From this perspective, both clinical trials and medical care are conceived as scientifically guided, therapeutically oriented activities conducted within the context of the physician-patient relationship."
—*New England Journal of Medicine*[5]

based medicine. The best evidence is found when all of these sources are properly considered, which this book attempts to do.

EVIDENCE-BASED PROOF FOR NATURAL REMEDIES

Each of the therapies discussed in this book is supported by legitimate studies. Most of these studies are prospective, which are the best kind of studies, as they measure what actually happens when specific remedies are given to subjects. Many of these studies are double-blind and placebo-controlled. Others are open trials, in which doctors, and sometimes patients, know which remedies are being given, and results are compared with migraine frequency before treatment. This book also contains individual case reports and series of cases. All of the studies and most of the case reports were published in medical journals after rigorous peer review. Each of these forms of information fits within the definition of evidence-based information.

As you will see, some of these natural remedies are equally effective or superior to many of the prescription drugs doctors commonly prescribe for migraines, and mainstream medical science is only beginning to accept this fact. In a review article published in 2005 that listed all of the proven effective methods of migraine prevention, five natural remedies (magnesium, riboflavin, coenzyme Q_{10}, butterbur, and feverfew) were mentioned alongside thirty-five pharmaceuticals.[6] In 2009, the Cochrane Collaboration—one of the most respected institutions in the world regarding medication therapy—published a huge review that compared studies of acupuncture for migraines. After examining twenty-two studies involving 4,419 subjects, the report concluded that "available studies suggest that acupuncture is at least as effective as, or possibly more effective than, prophylactic drug treatment, and has fewer adverse effects."[7]

Another large review of studies on migraine prevention found riboflavin and the herb feverfew to be as effective as the drugs gabapentin (Neurontin), verapamil (Calan), aspirin, naproxen (Aleve), and atenolol (Tenormin), which is similar to propranolol. Moreover, these natural remedies ranked superior for preventing migraines than amitriptyline (Elavil), diltiazem (Cardizem), ibuprofen (Motrin), and cyproheptadine (Periactin). The author of the review, Dr. C. Landy, stated:

> Nonpharmacologic treatments may be appropriate for patients who prefer such treatment, or for those who do not benefit from or are unable to take specific pharmacologic treatments because of poor tolerability, medical contraindications, pregnancy or nursing.[8]

This is a perfectly reasonable recommendation. The fact is that there is plenty of evidence-based proof supporting the use of natural remedies to stop migraines. If you are reading this book, you are already open to this idea. Perhaps someday the majority of doctors will be as well, which would allow them to discover the benefits of these natural therapies for themselves. As suggested in an article by R.W. Evans and F.R. Taylor:

> Many migraineurs are quite concerned about the toxicity of prescription medications and prefer alternative treatments regarded by them to be "natural" and thus relatively free of any side effects. If you (doctors) are knowledgeable about these treatments, patients are likely to perceive you to be an enlightened physician who understands and is sympathetic to their concerns and preferences.[9]

We all win when migraineurs are helped by natural remedies. Individual sufferers are relieved of the pain and limitations brought about by their migraines.

Doctors obtain the satisfaction of helping many while harming few. Health care costs drop dramatically, with fewer doctor and emergency room visits, and fewer pricey drugs.

At your next doctor's appointment, ask your physician if there are any natural treatments for migraines that might work for your condition. If you have read some impressive studies on natural treatments for migraine headaches, ask your doctor to look at the information with you. While you do not need your doctor's approval to try any of the remedies in this book, talking about the subject of natural therapies may broaden your physician's outlook, which may lead to more open-minded therapy options for other migraine patients. The mainstream medical attitude will change only from the ground up, because the drug industry and academic medicine tightly control medical school education and doctors' continuing education. So, gently, respectfully, offer what you've learned to your doctors. Tell them what has helped you. Some of your doctors may surprise you and show an interest. For the others, at least you have planted a seed that may grow if other patients do the same. In the meantime, you have done a good deed, and good deeds have a way of adding up. This is why I have written this book, and this is why you are reading it now.

It is said that the pen is mightier than the sword. Indeed it is, but only when people like you and I carry ideas such as these forward. I hope the following remedies help relieve your migraines and those of your loved ones, and make the medical system a little better and a little safer at the same time.

1. WHAT ARE MIGRAINES?

Although tension headaches are the most common type of headache, migraine headaches drive many more people to see a doctor. Most people get an occasional tension headache and assume that migraines are similar or perhaps a bit worse. In reality, migraines are an entirely different phenomenon, one that is often severe enough to be disabling.

The World Health Organization (WHO) ranks the discomfort of a migraine as one of the worst types of pain known to humans. As such, this affliction can have a profound impact on an individual's quality of life, sense of well-being, and ability to operate day to day. About 90 percent of sufferers report being functionally impaired during migraine attacks, and more than 50 percent report reduced capacity. Migraines result in 112 million bedridden days per year, at a cost of $13 billion in lost work productivity and over $1 billion in direct medical expenses annually.[1,2] Many migraine sufferers, also called *migraineurs*, cannot work due to their condition and endure substantial economic losses from their reduced income. They must also face the mounting costs of doctors' appointments and emergency room visits, medications, and medical tests. In addition, migraineurs are forced to live with the emotional strain that this disorder places on them, their families, and their social relationships. It is a problem that may impair the victim's daily life more than any other non-lethal chronic disease.

WHAT IS THE DEFINITION OF A MIGRAINE?

A migraine is generally defined as a headache that causes intense throbbing in one area of the head, most often above or behind one eye. A patient of mine once described it as "feeling like I've been stabbed in the eye." Migraines are often, but not always, accompanied by severe sensitivity to light and sound, and sufferers often have to retreat to a quiet and dark room before the pain gradually subsides over hours or days.

Preceding an attack, about a third of people with migraines experience symptoms known as *auras.* Auras are characterized by visual disturbances such as zigzag patterns, flashing lights, blind spots before the eyes, or double vision. Impairments of memory or thought, mood disturbances, or other signs of brain dysfunction may also occur.

Some doctors think that these symptoms must be evident to diagnose migraine disorder, but this belief is incorrect. Because many migraineurs do not have these symptoms, a diagnosis should be based on the nature and severity of their pain. In fact, the *New England Journal of Medicine* states that "any severe and recurrent headache is most likely to be a form of migraine and to be responsive to anti-migraine therapy."[3]

IS IT A REGULAR HEADACHE OR A MIGRAINE?

Migraines are often mistaken for other types of headaches. It is estimated that 75 percent of people who seek medical care for recurrent pain in the back of the head or neck, and 90 percent of those with recurrent sinus headaches are actually having migraines. Experts say that the condition should be suspected in any person with repeated disabling headaches.

Tension headaches usually occur along the sides of the head as a result of tightened muscles along the skull, while migraines most often appear in the frontal area above one or both eyes. Migraine attacks usually last four to seventy-two hours. While the average length of a migraine is twenty-four hours, they can last a week or more. While migraines are often accompanied by numerous other disturbances, such as those mentioned earlier, tension headaches are not usually associated with these secondary symptoms.

WHO GETS MIGRAINES?

According to neurologist and best-selling author Oliver Sacks, "Migraine affects a substantial minority of the population, occurs in all civilizations, and has been recognized since the dawn of recorded history. If it was a scourge to Caesar, Paul, Kant, and Freud, it is also a daily fact of life to anonymous millions who suffer in silence."[4] A brief list of others afflicted by this condition includes Thomas Jefferson, Virginia Woolf, Lewis Carroll, Friedrich Nietzsche, Peter Tchaikovsky, Alexander Graham Bell, Elvis Presley, and Elizabeth Taylor. Today, 20 million women and 8 million men suffer from migraines in the United States alone, and approximately 15 percent of all people will experience at least one migraine over a lifetime. These numbers may be deceiving, though, as they represent only those people who have been diagnosed with migraines. Countless others may go undocumented.

This disorder occurs predominantly in Caucasians and in people ages 25 to 55, after which the incidence drops. Still, in people over 60 years of age, migraines affect 8 percent of women and 3 percent of men. In this age bracket, however, migraines must be distinguished from transient ischemic attacks, also known as TIAs, which temporarily impair blood flow to the brain. They must also be differentiated from full-blown strokes. A key factor used to diagnose a stroke, in fact, is whether or not the patient has a history of migraines.[5]

Why are women afflicted with this problem almost three times as often as men? We simply do not know at this time. What is known is that genetics play a role in who gets migraines. An individual who has relatives with a history of migraines is 50 percent more likely to experience these headaches than someone without a familial connection to them. Personally, in my practice, I see similar familial tendencies in association with other conditions such as panic disorder and depression.

Children also experience migraines. Although other problems must be considered and ruled out, any severe headache that happens repeatedly in a child's life is probably a migraine. Interestingly, these headaches can occur in almost any part of a child's body. Any consistently debilitating pain marked by perfectly normal intervals between attacks may well be a migraine variant in a child, provided there are no positive findings from other medical tests.

WHAT CAUSES MIGRAINES?

There is an old saying in medicine that the more theories we have about a disease, the less we actually know about it. There are plenty of theories about the cause of migraine headaches, yet not one of them explains the disorder adequately. For decades, medical science has been seeking a basic underlying factor of migraines, but my view is that, with so many potential mechanisms, it is likely that these headaches arise in different people as a result of different underlying impairments. This is why this disorder varies so greatly in frequency, severity, intensity, triggers, auras, age of onset, and effective therapies. The many different possible processes involved in migraines include:

- Areas of depression spreading across the surface of the brain
- Erratic constriction and then dilation of blood vessels in the brain
- Excessive activation of platelets that release activating substances
- Excessive excitation in the brain or cranial nerves (trigeminal, occipital)
- Hyperactivity of the sympathetic nervous system
- Impaired metabolism or utilization of serotonin, dopamine, melatonin, prostaglandins, or arachidonic acid

- Impaired oxygen metabolism in mitochondria in the cells

- Inadequate oxygen concentrations in cells of nerves and blood vessels

- Inflammation of nerves and blood vessels

Because migraineurs are typically trouble-free between attacks, it was long believed that this condition did not cause permanent damage to the body. Today, many experts consider migraine disorder to be a chronic condition that can cause structural injuries. People who experience migraines with auras have been shown to have a slightly increased risk of stroke, while those without auras do not. The risk of stroke is also elevated in all migraine sufferers who smoke or take birth control pills.

WHAT TRIGGERS MIGRAINES?

In some people, migraines can be triggered by foods such as coffee, chocolate, alcohol, spices, salt, cheese, or food additives. Changes in sleep patterns or other biorhythms, or in ovulation or onset of menstruation, can also provoke this disorder. Other triggers include the scent of perfume, smoke from cigarettes or cigars, diesel or gasoline fumes, paint, stripes on the freeway, blaring music, changes in the weather, and medications such as nitroglycerin drugs and hormones. Finally, light is a trigger for approximately 50 percent of migraine victims.

HOW CAN MIGRAINES BE TREATED?

Mainstream treatment of migraine headaches almost always means prescription drugs. Unfortunately, there are just as many people who do not benefit from these drugs as those who do. And even those who do achieve positive results often have to deal with the unpleasant side effects of these medications—side effects so unpleasant or dangerous that they cause people to quit treatment. This book offers another approach—a medically valid, scientifically proven, and safer approach that can help people with migraines just as effectively (indeed, sometimes more effectively), and with fewer adverse effects, than prescription drugs.

2. BIOIDENTICAL REMEDIES

A bioidentical supplement is molecularly identical to a substance that is present in the human body. Because a bioidentical remedy has the same chemical structure as the natural compound, the body recognizes it and reacts to it as normal. In contrast, pharmaceuticals, herbs, and even some foods can cause significant side effects when the body reacts to them as foreign substances. Bioidentical migraine remedies include supplements such as riboflavin (a vitamin normally found in certain foods), melatonin (a naturally occurring hormone), and magnesium (an essential dietary mineral).

RIBOFLAVIN

Riboflavin, also known as vitamin B_2, is a member of the B family of vitamins, which are essential for preserving health in humans and animals. The term riboflavin is a combination of *ribose*, a type of sugar that forms part of riboflavin's structure, and *flavin*, the component that produces vitamin's yellow color. Isolated in 1879, this nutrient plays a key role in converting food into energy, facilitating enzymatic activity, and using dietary protein to build new cells and tissues.[1, 2, 3, 4, 5] Riboflavin also serves as an antioxidant, neutralizing the destructive substances known as free radicals, which damage DNA. Finally, it assists in the conversion of other B vitamins, such as pyridoxine (vitamin B_6) and folate (vitamin B_9), into their active forms.

Like all B vitamins, riboflavin is soluble in water and absorbed quickly upon ingestion. It is stored only in small amounts in the body and eliminated via the urine. The Recommended Daily Intake (RDI) of riboflavin for both men and women is 1.2 mg a day. People who eat healthy, balanced diets usually obtain adequate riboflavin from food. Items high in ribo-flavin include milk, cheese, yogurt, broccoli, spinach, turnip greens, asparagus, bananas, beef, pork, chicken, and enriched grains.

How It Works

One current theory suggests that migraines occur because of a dysfunction in oxygen metabolism in the mitochondria of nerve cells. Mitochondria are often referred to as the power plants of cells. By improving mitochondrial function, riboflavin boosts the energy production of cells. This action may be the reason behind this vitamin's ability to halt migraines. Perhaps not coincidentally, coenzyme Q_{10}, another natu-ral migraine remedy, has also been shown to improve mitochondrial function.

Scientific Reports of Riboflavin's Effectiveness

After first being synthesized in 1935, it wasn't long before medical science discovered riboflavin's effectiveness in the treatment of migraines. Over the years, there have been numerous reports of this vitamin's ability to stop acute migraines and prevent them from happening in the future.

● **1946 (First Report).** Impressed by reports of the successful use of riboflavin in the treatment of other disorders, Dr. Clifford Smith of Montreal started two of his migraine patients on this vitamin. According to his findings, "the results from the first were more than significant."[6] He then widened his study to include another nineteen patients—fifteen women and four men. These people had suffered migraines for two to ten years or longer. Dr. Smith prescribed 10 mg per day of riboflavin. Upon learning that this dosage was inadequate, he increased it to 5 mg, three times a day. In most patients, migraine symptoms diminished over several months of continued riboflavin use. Some subjects found that hourly doses would stop acute migraine attacks. (See "Natural Remedies for Acute Migraines" on page 117.) Of the nineteen subjects, eighteen obtained complete cessation of migraines or marked improvement with continued riboflavin therapy over several months. Even the one remaining patient, who did not take riboflavin regularly, experienced modest improvement.

● **1994.** A study conducted in Belgium by Dr. J. Schoenen and associates demonstrated that 400 mg of riboflavin per day was "an effective, low-cost prophylactic treatment for migraine devoid of short-term side effects."[7] In the month before riboflavin therapy, the forty-nine subjects averaged 8.7 migraine attacks—in essence, more than two migraines a week, or one migraine every 3.5 days. In the final month of taking 400 mg of riboflavin with breakfast, the forty-nine subjects averaged 2.9 migraine attacks, less than one a week, or one migraine every nine days. These results indicated a 60-percent reduction in the frequency of migraine episodes. The improvement was not limited to a few subjects, but instead was shared by most of them. Indeed, forty of the forty-nine (79 percent) riboflavin users experienced a decrease in migraine frequency of at least 50 percent.

In addition to lowering the occurrence of migraines, riboflavin also reduced their severity by nearly 70 percent on average among the subjects during the final month of therapy. This result was highly significant. "On average, the migraine severity score decreased in the entire group of patients after treatment," the authors explained. When the researchers measured the comprehensive effect of treatment, they found an astonishing 68-percent overall improvement after three months of treatment. In several patients, migraine attacks stopped altogether. This result equals or exceeds the improvement seen with most prescription migraine medications today.

● **1998.** Building on their 1994 work, Dr. J. Schoenen and associates undertook a more rigorous scientific study that was double-blind, randomized, and placebo-controlled.[8] It involved fifty-five subjects, more than 75 percent of whom were women. One group of subjects received a placebo while the other received 400 mg of riboflavin daily with breakfast for three months. The participants had experienced approximately four migraines a month for an average of thirteen years (ranging from one to forty-seven years). Subjects' ages averaged thirty-six years (ranging from eighteen to sixty-two years), and they had encountered migraines that lasted an average of thirty-four hours (ranging from six hours to three and a half days) per month. The study measured the effectiveness, if any, of riboflavin on migraine attack frequency, duration, and severity.

The results of the research were impressive. By the end of the study, the frequency of migraine attacks dropped approximately 50 percent in the riboflavin group. In comparison, the placebo group experienced an increase in migraines. In the riboflavin group, 59 percent of subjects benefited from a significant reduction in the duration of migraines, while only 15 percent of the placebo group experienced similar improvement. Severity was also decreased with the use of riboflavin. By the end of the study, subjects in the riboflavin group obtained a 68-percent reduction in migraine severity compared with the group that received a placebo. All of these findings were statistically significant.

Best results were obtained in the third and final month of therapy, indicating that it takes time for the body to use riboflavin maximally in the reduction of migraines. It is possible that an extended use of riboflavin might have delivered even better results. Notably, people in the riboflavin group took their pills reliably, much more so than in similar studies involving prescription drugs. This is likely due to the fact that side effects were few. There were actually only two mild side effects—heartburn and loose bowel movements—in the riboflavin subjects. The authors of the study concluded, "This randomized controlled trial demonstrates that a daily oral dose of 400 mg riboflavin is significantly superior to placebo for migraine prophylaxis." Once again, riboflavin's ability to prevent migraines was proven.

● **2004.** The effectiveness of riboflavin in the prevention of migraines was investigated by Dr. C. Boehnke and associates in an open-label study at a specialty clinic for migraine patients who had not responded to drug therapy.[9] Twenty-three people (82 percent of whom were women) were experiencing two to eight migraines per month. Their ages averaged fifty-two years (ranging from twenty to sixty-five years). The main measurement for riboflavin's effectiveness was a reduction in migraine frequency. In the month prior to riboflavin therapy, the patients averaged four migraine attacks. After three months of riboflavin therapy, the frequency of attacks was reduced to two migraine attacks per month, amounting to a 50-percent improvement. This reduction was maintained until the end of the study three months later. During this time, the necessity for acute migraine medication (a triptan drug or pain medication) dropped by 35.7 percent in the riboflavin group. Moreover, in the month prior to riboflavin treatment, the average migraine attack duration was 50 hours. After six months of taking riboflavin, the average attack duration was 28 hours—a decrease of 44 percent. Although headache intensity showed no improvement with riboflavin, the results of this research were statistically significant.

In regard to adverse side effects, three patients (10 percent of the group) developed mild symptoms such as stomach pain, diarrhea, and redness of the face. In comparison, prescription drugs for migraines frequently cause adverse side effects, some serious, in 30 percent of patients.[10] The authors of this study concluded, "In line with previous studies, our findings show that riboflavin is a safe and well-tolerated alternative in migraine prophylaxis. . . . We propose riboflavin as an alternative choice for prophylactic anti-migraine treatment."

● **2009.** Forty-one children and adolescents participated in a study of riboflavin's effectiveness in preventing their chronic migraines. Significant reductions in migraine frequency and intensity were seen with 200 mg and 400 mg doses of riboflavin per day.[11] (See "Preventing Migraines in Children and Adolescents" on page 107.)

Additional Evidence

As mentioned earlier, a 2004 review of studies on migraine prevention noted riboflavin to be as effective as the pharmaceuticals gabapentin (Neurontin), atenolol (Tenormin), verapamil (Calan), aspirin, and naproxen (Aleve); and superior to amitriptyline (Elavil), diltiazem (Cardizem), ibuprofen (Motrin), and cyproheptadine (Periactin).[12] Additionally, of the thirty-five effective migraine therapies listed in a 2005

review, riboflavin was among the five natural remedies.[13] Finally, the online resource The People's Pharmacy (www.peoplespharmacy.com) posted anecdotal
reports of riboflavin's effectiveness in 2008 and 2009.
The first one stated:

> I had headaches for over 30 years—migraine, ten-
> sion, cluster, you name it! The health clinic told me
> to take mega doses of vitamin B_2 and no pain-
> killers. I learned I had been causing headaches
> because of a rebound effect from pain killers. My
> headaches stopped in less than 30 days and I have
> been headache-free for more than a decade. The
> vitamin costs me $7 for 100 tablets.[14]

The second account was just as compelling:

> Thank you for writing about taking vitamin B_2 on a
> daily basis to prevent migraine headaches. I have
> suffered from them for 17 years and have seen too
> many medical doctors including two neurologists,
> two ear, nose and throat doctors, and an acupunc-
> turist. I had sinus scans and have tried many med-
> ications that never worked. I started taking the
> vitamin B_2 and I couldn't believe how much it
> helped. I may get an occasional headache now,
> once a month if that. I used to get a couple every
> week. I am thrilled to finally be free of headaches
> for the most part and have told my doctor to please
> share this with other patients with frequent
> migraine headaches.[15]

These personal stories are important and worth
taking seriously. Case reports are valuable sources of
information in this age of evidence-based medicine.

What the Research Tells Us

Riboflavin has been proven effective for reducing the frequency and duration of migraine headaches in four different studies. Migraine intensity was also reduced in three studies. The results of this research were highly significant scientifically. Yet, more than six decades after the first report of riboflavin's effectiveness, few doctors have any knowledge about using this vitamin in migraine treatment. Do we need any further proof of the deficiencies in medical education and the way in which the drug industry dominates treatment decisions?

Migraines can be difficult to treat successfully. Many migraine sufferers do not respond to prescription drugs or are unable to take then because of the medication's intolerable side effects. Riboflavin, however, has been shown to work in a high percentage of people with intractable migraines, and with fewer and milder side effects. In addition, riboflavin is not known to cause dangerous interactions with the other medications you may be taking. Riboflavin will cost you less than ten dollars for one hundred pills. If this vitamin replaced prescription drugs for only 10 percent of migraine sufferers, it would save medical centers, hospitals, insurance companies, and governments millions of dollars.

Dosage

You may obtain the best results by using 400 mg of riboflavin daily. If you respond favorably, you may continue treatment indefinitely. This vitamin's impact on migraine frequency, duration, and intensity sometimes occurs quickly, but reports indicate that maximum benefit may not be seen until three or four months of therapy.

For the tiny number of people who have adverse effects with riboflavin, a lower dose of 200 mg per day can be used, and even lower doses may be tried. Splitting the optimal riboflavin dosage into 200 mg at breakfast and dinner may also reduce the occurrence of side effects. The one change you will definitely notice with riboflavin is an iridescent yellow urine color, which is harmless.

COENZYME Q$_{10}$

Coenzyme Q$_{10}$ (CoQ$_{10}$), also known as ubiquinone, is a naturally occurring substance that has many uses in the human body, the primary of which is energy production. CoQ$_{10}$ deficiencies have been identified in patients with many disorders, including cardiovascular disease, diabetes, Parkinson's and Alzheimer's diseases, liver and kidney disorders, cancer, and even migraines.

How It Works

Migraines may be caused by abnormal oxygen metabolism in the mitochondria of nerve cells. CoQ$_{10}$ is needed for normal mitochondrial function and the production of energy in the mitochondria of cells. CoQ$_{10}$ is similar to riboflavin in this regard. And like riboflavin, it improves cellular energy production and seems to prevent migraines. CoQ$_{10}$ is also a potent antioxidant and may reduce the release of inflammatory free radicals, which are associated with migraines.

Because of its antioxidant properties and ability to revitalize mitochondrial function, CoQ_{10} has even proven beneficial for people with certain heart, muscle, and nerve dysfunctions.[16]

Scientific Reports of Coenzyme Q_{10}'s Effectiveness

While the effectiveness of coenzyme Q_{10} in the treatment of migraine headaches has only begun to be studied, the three reports published on the subject over the last decade paint a very optimistic picture.

● **2002 (First Report).** The first inquiry into whether CoQ_{10} might help prevent migraine headaches involved twenty-six women and six men, all with long histories of migraines.[17] The frequency of their migraines averaged between two and eight attacks per month. The study was open-label, meaning that the subjects knew they were receiving CoQ_{10}. The dosage used was 150 mg per day.

Most patients improved to some degree with CoQ_{10} treatment, with 94 percent of subjects obtaining at least a 25-percent reduction in the number of days with migraine per month. More impressively, 61 percent (nearly two-thirds!) of the subjects experienced a 50-percent or greater decrease in the number of days with migraine. In some individual cases, the decrease in the number of days with migraine per month was outstanding, as shown in the table on the following page.

During the one-month baseline phase of the study, in which no treatment was given, subjects averaged

Subject Number	Baseline (Number of Days with Migraine in One-Month Period Before Treatment)	Number of Days with Migraine in One-Month Period after CoQ$_{10}$ Treatment	Improvement
2	9.0	2.4	73 %
8	8.6	2.0	87 %
15	7.5	0.8	89 %
24	10.8	1.5	86 %
26	8.2	0.7	92 %
31	8.8	2.5	72 %

4.9 migraines. In the third month of CoQ$_{10}$ therapy, migraine frequency dropped to an average of 2.8—an improvement of 43 percent. Moreover, during the baseline phase of the study, the patients averaged 7.3 days with migraines. During the third month of CoQ$_{10}$ therapy, they averaged only three days with migraines— an improvement of 60 percent. This means that the migraines were not only fewer in number, but also shorter in duration.

In addition, the effectiveness of CoQ$_{10}$ increased with each subsequent month of treatment. Over the first month of CoQ$_{10}$ treatment, migraine frequency decreased by only 13 percent. Yet, by the end of the third month, average migraine occurrence displayed a 55-percent drop. Only one subject experienced a slight increase in migraines, and only two subjects did not show any improvement with CoQ$_{10}$. Most participants, however, did not see a decrease in migraine severity with CoQ$_{10}$ treatment. Overall, the results with CoQ_{10} exceeded those obtained with most pre-scription drugs used for migraines. And no side effects were reported.

This study leaves some unanswered questions. Would sixth months or a year of CoQ_{10} therapy provide even better results? Additionally, the dosage of 150 mg is less than used by many alternative doctors for other disorders, such as heart failure. Would higher dosages, such as 300 mg per day (100 mg three times a day) provide even greater reductions in migraine frequency and duration? The researchers aptly summarized their findings by stating, "Coenzyme Q_{10} looks to be an excellent choice for initial therapy for prevention of episodic migraine if confirmed by controlled studies of efficacy. It can be given to almost any age group without fear of significant side effects." Note that the doctors recommended CoQ_{10} as an "initial therapy," meaning before drugs or other supplements.

● **2005.** Forty-two chronic migraine sufferers, ages eighteen to sixty-five, were studied in a double-blind, randomized, placebo-controlled study.[18] The subjects had experienced migraines for at least one year (some for over thirty years), sustaining three to eight migraines per month. Eighty percent of the subjects were women. After three months without any preventive treatment for their migraines, the subjects received either 100 mg of CoQ_{10} three times daily or a placebo for three months.

In the final month of treatment, patients taking CoQ_{10} obtained greater reductions in migraine frequency and total number of days with migraine than those taking the placebo. For example, only 14 percent of the placebo group obtained a 50-percent or greater reduction in migraine frequency. Yet, 48 percent of CoQ_{10} subjects experienced a 50-percent or greater decrease in migraine frequency. These results were statistically significant.

Those taking CoQ_{10} saw further improvement in migraine frequency with each subsequent month of treatment. The researchers commented on this phenomenon by stating, "The effect of CoQ_{10} seems to begin after the first month and to be maximal after 3 months." Since the treatment phase of the study was only three months in length, it is possible that the benefits of CoQ_{10} might have continued to grow with additional months of therapy.

Although CoQ_{10} markedly reduced the occurrence of migraine headaches, it did not impact their severity or duration in this study. Only one adverse effect was noted in the group—a skin allergy. The researchers suggested that because of CoQ_{10}'s low risk and high degree of tolerability, it might also be considered for use in pregnant women, and advised further study of this possibility.

● **2007.** In a study of 252 children and adolescents, 46 percent of subjects taking CoQ_{10} saw a 50-percent or greater reduction in migraine frequency.[19] Others obtained lesser degrees of improvement. (See "Preventing Migraines in Children and Adolescents" on page 107.)

What the Research Tells Us

The research demonstrates that coenzyme Q_{10} is an effective and safe natural remedy for migraine headaches in a high percentage of patients. CoQ_{10} is most useful in reducing headache frequency and the total number of days per month that migraines occur. It does not appear, however, to decrease migraine intensity.

CoQ_{10} is very well tolerated. An abundance of research involving other medical disorders has been done with this substance, and they show that it causes few side effects. Most common symptoms are gastric upset or nausea, which occurred in less than 1 percent of subjects in these studies.

Dosage

Considering CoQ_{10}'s effectiveness and low risk, you can consider this remedy a first-line treatment for migraines. You can start with 150 mg a day, increasing the dosage to 100 mg three times a day, if required.

MAGNESIUM

Magnesium is one of the most important elements in the human body. This mineral plays a vital role in healthy muscle and nerve function, heart rhythm, immune system function, and bone strength. Despite a vast medical literature on magnesium, and its frequent use in the prevention of cardiac arrhythmias and the treatment of seizures from eclampsia, most doctors know little about magnesium's ability to combat a number of other health conditions. In contrast, magnesium is one of alternative doctors' most prescribed remedies.

How It Works

As one of the most common minerals in the human
body, magnesium participates in hundreds of biochemical reactions within cells. Moreover, it governs
smooth muscle activity in the arteries and nerve
activity in the nervous system. Both of these are
major factors in the development of migraines. Ani-
mal and human studies have repeatedly demonstrated that low levels of magnesium can lead to
spasms of the cerebral arteries, which are involved in
migraine headaches.

The majority of people in western countries lack
the proper amount of magnesium. Surveys reveal that
70 to 80 percent of the populations of France and the
United States are magnesium deficient. This is generally attributed to changes in eating habits over the last
century, depletion of soil, and the mass production of
refined foods, which lack magnesium. Equally important, it has also been proven that people with low levels
of magnesium incur a higher incidence of migraines.

Scientific Reports of Magnesium's Effectiveness

Human studies have shown magnesium to be an
effective therapy for a variety of disorders, including
asthma, cardiac arrhythmias, high blood pressure,
muscle cramps, pain syndromes, Raynaud's phenomenon, and migraines. In fact, research on magnesium's
ability to treat migraines dates back almost a century.

● **1933 (First Report).** In an article published by the
medical journal *Lancet*, authors described the

response of a patient with severe migraines to treatment with magnesium:

> A married woman, 32 years old, had nocturnal attacks of severe headache with vomiting and palpitation. I had the opportunity of witnessing an actual attack and I realised [sic] that I was dealing with a case of real migraine. A dozen injections of magnesium sulphate cut short the attacks and she now has been free from them for a year.[20]

While the method of injection and the dosage of magnesium were not detailed, the prolonged absence of further migraines may be explained by increased cellular levels of magnesium following the dozen treatments.

● **1995.** A study that used 1,000 mg of intravenous magnesium to halt acute migraines proved highly successful.[21, 22, 23] Two additional studies—one in 2001 and another in 2002—also demonstrated magnesium's effectiveness in stopping migraines already in progress. (For further information on the research into magnesium as a treatment for acute migraines, see "Natural Remedies for Acute Migraines" on page 117.)

● **1996.** Eighty-one migraine patients between the ages of eighteen and sixty-five were given magnesium (trimagnesium citrate) as treatment for their long-term migraines.[24] Prior to treatment, the group averaged 3.6 migraines per month. A baseline was established by a four-week phase without therapy, after which some subjects received 600 mg of magnesium orally every day for twelve weeks, while others received a placebo. Treatment with magnesium showed progressive reductions in migraine frequency. During the final month of therapy, occurrence of migraine headaches was reduced by 42 percent on average in the magnesium group. The placebo group, however, experienced a decrease of only 16 percent. The result with magnesium was statistically significant, as the following table shows.

In addition, the number of days with migraines

Length of Study	Average Number of Migraines in One-Month Period: Magnesium Group	Average Number of Migraines in One-Month Period: Placebo Group
Baseline	3.7	3.7
At Four Weeks	3.3	3.9
At Eight Weeks	2.7	3.5
At Twelve Weeks	2.2	3.3

was significantly reduced in the magnesium group versus the placebo group, as was the amount of pain medication used. Magnesium therapy also yielded greater reductions in migraine duration and intensity compared to placebo. While improvement with magnesium therapy was seen after four weeks, maximum benefit was obtained at twelve weeks. Even greater results may have been seen if the study had been extended another twelve weeks.

Adverse effects occurred with both magnesium and placebo. Magnesium can cause diarrhea, which occurred in 19 percent of the magnesium group. General gastric irritation was seen in 5 percent of the magnesium group.

Contrasting this research was an additional double-blind, randomized, placebo-controlled study published a few months later.[25] In this study, magnesium therapy provided a 50-percent reduction in migraine duration in only 29 percent of users, which was the same percentage that responded to placebo. There were also no differences between magnesium therapy and placebo when it came to lowering migraine intensity or frequency. Side effects were common with magnesium, including five subjects who had soft stools, five who had diarrhea, and three who experienced palpitations. Eight of the placebo subjects reported side effects.

This study proved that magnesium did not work and caused many side effects, right? Not necessarily so. The type of magnesium researched in this study is used primarily in horses, not humans. It is called MAH, magnesium aspartate hydrochloride. The fact that many of the research subjects developed loose stools or diarrhea with this form of magnesium indicates that it was poorly absorbed and was instead carried to the large bowel. Poor absorption means low blood levels, which means inadequate response to therapy.

In the first 1996 study, in which magnesium was proven to be highly effective against migraines, the authors used trimagnesium citrate, a better grade of magnesium that is well absorbed. This would explain why this research demonstrated numerous positive results and few adverse effects, whereas the second study showed the opposite.

● **2008.** The authors of a double-blind, randomized, placebo-controlled study sought to determine whether some types of migraines would be more responsive to magnesium therapy than others.[26] They tested subjects who experienced migraines without aura symptoms, treating them with 600 mg of magnesium citrate (a superior grade of magnesium) per day. The response to therapy was evaluated by both clinical assessment and sophisticated visual and cerebral testing. Overall, magnesium treatment produced statistically significant reductions in migraine frequency and severity compared to baseline levels and placebo treatment.

Additional Evidence

An individual's experience using magnesium to treat migraines was posted on the online resource The People's Pharmacy. The subject reported:

> I used to suffer with migraines so bad that I had a kit to give myself shots. I could never bring myself to give myself a shot. I had heard about magnesium being good for migraines, so I thought what can it hurt to try it? I have taken it for years now and NO MIGRAINES!! It truly worked for me.[27]

A second testimonial comes from the author of this book. I used to get intermittent yet severe migraines. Not knowing the connection between migraines and magnesium therapy, I began taking magnesium for a separate medical condition. A year later, I realized I hadn't had any migraines, and over the past decade have experienced only a handful of mild headaches.

What the Research Tells Us

My experience with magnesium is this: When it works, it works well. It may be that, as mentioned earlier, people with magnesium deficiencies are highly responsive to magnesium therapy, while those with normal amounts of magnesium benefit less from this type of treatment. Unfortunately, it is not a simple matter to differentiate people with magnesium deficiencies from those with adequate levels of this mineral. Laboratory testing is highly inaccurate, so the most reliable test is to simply take magnesium and see if it works.

As a mineral that is natural to be human body, magnesium is very safe. Indeed, it is a routine therapy in cardiac intensive care units and maternal intensive care units. When used properly in these units or in emergency rooms, magnesium is low risk and has few adverse effects. Using magnesium therapeutically can be difficult, however, because some of the commonly used forms of magnesium—such as magnesium oxide—are poorly absorbed and often cause diarrhea. Milk of Magnesia is the prototype of a magnesium laxative. Yet, some doctors still recommend it, thinking it is a good source of magnesium. It is not, because the body does not absorb it.

Magnesium amino acid complexes, also known as chelates (pronounced *kee-lates*), are a better form of magnesium. These include magnesium citrate, lactate, and malate. I have personally found success with a product that combines magnesium amino acid chelate with a small amount of protein. When I first tried magnesium, I was unable to tolerate it in any other form, and for over a decade I have been using this configuration with great results. Even so, some people cannot tolerate most magnesium pills, and in such cases I recommend magnesium chloride crystals that can be dissolved in water. I usually have patients take it before bedtime. If side effects occur, I recommend splitting the dosage, taking half in the morning and half in the evening.

Dosage

Start with a low dosage of magnesium such as 100 mg twice daily. The dosage can be gradually increased to the Recommended Daily Intake for adults, which is 400 mg per day. Be sure to drink ample liquids. Dosing should be done cautiously in seniors and those with impaired kidney function.

Alternative doctors may prescribe higher dosages of magnesium for stubborn conditions. Amounts of 600 to 800 mg per day are commonly prescribed. Several of the studies listed in this chapter used 600 mg per day. Your magnesium blood level should be checked after a few months of use, but toxicity is rare in people with normal kidney function and adequate hydration. Symptoms of magnesium toxicity include weakness, slow heartbeat or reflexes, or drowsiness. As is the case with any supplement, it takes time for magnesium to show significant effects. Although some decrease in migraine frequency and duration may be seen within a month, maximum improvement usually requires three to six months of therapy.

MELATONIN

Isolated in 1958, melatonin (N-acetyl-5-methoxytryptamine) is a sleep-promoting hormone that is naturally produced by the body. It is synthesized by a small gland located beneath the center of the brain called the pineal gland. The creation of melatonin is stimulated by darkness and inhibited by light. In fact, there is currently some concern that watching television or using a computer in the evening may suppress the production of melatonin and delay sleep due to the light from the screen. On the other hand, people have used television for decades as a way of facilitating sleep.

Over recent decades, altered melatonin levels have been identified in people with migraine headaches, menstrual migraines, and chronic migraine disorders.[28,29,30] These findings suggest that treatment with this hormone may aid in migraine prevention.

How It Works

Melatonin has a multitude of effects on humans. In addition to its sleep-promoting functions, melatonin has anti-inflammatory properties, scavenges free radicals, and suppresses the production of substances that promote pain. It also influences the interactions between nerves and blood vessels, and modulates serotonin activity.[31,32]

It is hypothesized that an imbalance in the relationship between the hypothalamus and pineal gland may lead to an inadequate release of melatonin. This, in turn, may underlie the occurrence of migraines in some people.[33]

Scientific Reports of Melatonin's Effectiveness

Although this chapter provides only two studies documenting the effectiveness of melatonin in migraine prevention, the reports are impressive and prove this hormone worthy of its place on the list of remedies.

• **2004 (First Report).** Thirty-four adult migraine patients—twenty-nine women and five men—were treated with a daily dose of 3 mg of melatonin for three months.[34] This was an open-label study in which the patients and doctors knew that melatonin was the treatment being administered. The patients' response to melatonin was compared to the frequency, intensity, and duration of their migraines during the one-month preliminary phase of the trial, during which no treatment was given.

Prior to the experiment, the study's participants were experiencing two to eight migraines per month. Of the thirty-two subjects who finished the study, twenty-five (80 percent!) obtained a 50-percent or greater reduction in migraine frequency. Migraine attacks stopped entirely in eight of the patients (25 percent). Another seven patients gained a 75-percent decrease in migraine attacks, while an additional ten patients obtained a reduction of 50 to 74 percent.

On average, melatonin therapy decreased headache occurrence by 60 percent, from almost eight migraines per month at baseline to three per month with treatment. In addition, migraine intensity dropped 25 percent, while migraine duration fell nearly 50 percent. All of these results were clinically significant.

A small degree of improvement was seen after one month of melatonin use, and this result increased consistently through the third month of therapy. Of those who did not improve with melatonin supplementation, none experienced an increase in migraine frequency.

Two people withdrew from the study—one due to excessive sedation and the other because of perceived hair loss. Interestingly, three of the people who completed the study also noted an increase in libido.

The findings of this study are impressive. Eighty percent of patients with a history of migraines obtained substantial reductions in migraine frequency, intensity, and duration.

● **2008.** Twenty-two children and adolescents participated in this study of melatonin as a treatment for chronic migraines. Impressive reductions in migraine frequency and intensity were seen with doses of 3 mg of melatonin at bedtime.[35] Of fourteen children and adolescents with migraines, ten (71 percent) obtained a reduction in migraine frequency of greater than 50 percent. (A full description of this study can be found in "Preventing Migraines in Children and Adolescents" on page 107.)

What the Research Tells Us

These reports show that melatonin therapy yields superior results to many of the commonly prescribed migraine drugs. Melatonin also has far fewer and milder adverse reactions. The most common side effect with melatonin is sedation. This is not a true side effect, however, as melatonin is normally produced by the body to facilitate sleep. In light of this fact, melatonin should always be taken before bedtime.

Dosage

The effective melatonin dosage can differ widely from person to person. If you are sensitive to medicinal substances, start with a low dosage. Melatonin supplements come in dosages of 0.5, 1, 2, 3, or 5 mg. They can be purchased in a fast-acting sublingual form (dissolved under the tongue) or a long-lasting sustained-release form. Only people who are ready to go to bed immediately should use sublingual melatonin. This type of melatonin may also be tried to halt acute migraines.

Long-lasting sustained-release melatonin might be helpful for people who awaken a few hours after taking standard melatonin. In certain individuals, however, sustained-release melatonin may cause morning grogginess. An alternative doctor can help you identify the best dosage and type of melatonin for your system.

5-HYDROXYTRYPTOPHAN (5-HTP)

5-hydroxytryptophan, also called 5-HTP, is an essential building block in the body's synthesis of serotonin, a neurotransmitter that facilitates communication between cells throughout the body. It is produced from the amino acid tryptophan, which is available in many foods.

How It Works

The chemical 5-HTP is converted into serotonin in the body. An increased level of 5-HTP results in an elevated amount of serotonin. Large concentrations of serotonin are found in the nervous system and gastrointestinal system. It is involved in the conduction of pain, and in the dilation and constriction of blood vessels, both of which play a role in the occurrence of migraines. It has been shown to promote vasodilation (dilation of blood vessels) in some people and vasoconstriction (constriction of blood vessels) in others. This fact may explain why 5-HTP prevents migraines for some people, but has no such effect on others.

The serotonin system is complicated. This fact is made clear when you consider that the herbs feverfew (see "Feverfew" on page 67) and white willow (see "White Willow" on page 74) can prevent migraines in many people by blocking serotonin activity, while 5-HTP, which encourages serotonin production, can also remedy these headaches. You might wonder how this can be. The answer is that there are many serotonin receptors throughout the body, and various therapies impact different serotonin receptors. So, while the activity of these substances may seem to contradict each other, they each can be effective migraine treatments.

Scientific Reports of 5-HTP's Effectiveness

The first report of the successful use of 5-HTP for preventing migraines was published in 1973. Despite the publication of additional positive studies over the past few decades, the medical establishment still hasn't adopted 5-HTP as an effective alternative therapy for migraine patients. The following reports explain why you should.

● **1973 (First Report).** In the April 1973 issue of *Headache*, Dr. Federigo Sicuteri reported the results of his study comparing 5-HTP and methysergide, a prescription drug proven to prevent migraines.[36] In the twenty subjects who took 1 mg of methysergide twice a day, migraine frequency during the forty-day period dropped from an average of 4.7 episodes before treatment to 2.3 episodes with therapy, a 55-percent improvement. In the twenty subjects who received 200 mg of 5-HTP once a day, migraine occurrence fell from an average of 4.5 to 2.1 episodes, a 55-percent improvement. The results of 5-HTP treatment were statistically significant and as impressive as those of methysergide therapy and many other drugs prescribed to prevent migraines.

Subjects that continued to take 5-HTP for four months saw the benefits of this substance persist. Dr. Sicuteri commented, "[5-HTP] appears to improve migraine in the same extent of the classic migraine prophylactic methysergide. The improvement is gradual and reaches the maximum after 2–3 weeks." Due to its many serious side effects, methysergide is not often prescribed to migraine patients today. 5-HTP, however, is natural to the body and causes few, if any, side effects. Those side effects that may occur are mild, and commonly include sedation, so it is best to take 5-HTP at night. In relation to sleep, another minor side effect is weird dreams.

• **1981.** Ranging from twenty-two to fifty-five years old, fifty-four women and six men participated in this study, which compared the benefits of aspirin to those of 5-HTP in the prevention of migraines.[37] The subjects had long histories of migraine headaches, lasting from five to thirty-five years, and their previous medication, pizotifen or methysergide, had not worked or had lost its effectiveness.

After a two-month period without any treatment, subjects were treated with either 5-HTP or aspirin for two months. Of the subjects who received a high dose of 5-HTP—1.5 grams per day—thirty-five of them completed the study. Twenty other subjects were given 2 g of aspirin per day.

The main measurement in this study was pain intensity. After taking 5-HTP for two months, seven of the thirty-five patients (20 percent) obtained a 100-percent improvement in pain intensity. Another fifteen subjects (43 percent) experienced improvement of 50 percent or greater, and nine (26 percent) saw benefits of less than 50 percent. Only four subjects (11 percent) did not improve.

Thus, twenty-two subjects (63 percent) obtained a 50-percent or greater reduction in their migraine

Number of 5-HTP Subjects	Improvement
7	100 %
15	≥ 50 %
9	< 50 %
4	0 %

pain, a result that exceeds most prescription remedies. Additionally, many 5-HTP patients saw a decrease in the duration of migraines. In contrast, the aspirin group obtained some initial benefits, which disappeared after a month.

Five people withdrew from the study, citing stomach upset due to 5-HTP. Gastrointestinal side effects with 5-HTP are infrequent and, in this study, were probably due to the high dosage used. Typically, dosages of 5-HTP range from 100 to 400 mg per day.

● **1984.** Dr. Giorgio Bono and colleagues studied the effects of 300 mg per day of 5-HTP in 100 people, ranging from twenty to sixty years old. The subjects suffered from various types of severe headaches and included eighty-four migraine victims. After four months of treatment, seventy-four people experienced a 60-percent or greater reduction in total pain scores. This was an excellent result. And although headache frequency did not improve statistically, substantial decreases in headache duration and intensity were seen.[38]

● **1985.** This double-blind crossover study involved thirty people with chronic headaches, including sixteen with migraines.[39] Treatment consisted of 400 mg of 5-HTP or a placebo every day for two months. Both 5-HTP and the placebo produced a reduction in headache frequency and severity, but the reduction was greater with 5-HTP.

Of the 5-HTP subjects, 48 percent obtained a 50-percent or greater decrease in headache symptoms—a good result. Adverse effects occurred in only six subjects and were mild and brief. The researchers stated, "We conclude that 5-HTP is a medication of moderate efficacy and remarkable safety, providing us with another alternative approach to chronic primary headache prophylaxis."

● **1986.** In this randomized and controlled study of migraine prevention, 124 subjects received either 600 mg of 5-HTP or 3 mg of the drug methysergide on a daily basis.[40] Methysergide was an effective and commonly used migraine drug at the time, but it is rarely used today because of serious side effects. The dosages used in this study were considerably higher than those used in the 1973 Sicuteri study described earlier.

Improvement was defined by the researchers as a reduction in migraine frequency or severity of 50 percent or greater. Treatment with 5-HTP resulted in significant improvements in 71 percent of subjects, while methysergide yielded a similar benefits in 75 percent of subjects. Therefore, the results of both therapies were virtually the same.

Compared with those who received a placebo, the improvements seen with both 5-HTP and methysergide treatments were statistically significant. Treatment with 5-HTP was most effective in reducing migraine severity and duration, but not migraine frequency.

Side effects from methysergide caused five subjects to quit treatment, whereas not one of the 5-HTP patients discontinued the study. Although the benefits seen with methysergide and 5-HTP were similar, 5-HTP was better tolerated and much safer than the alternative.

● **1991.** In a double-blind study, thirty-nine subjects with chronic migraines were given either 5-HTP or propranolol, a commonly prescribed medication for migraine prevention.[41] Both 5-HTP and propranolol produced statistically significant reductions in migraine frequency, although propranolol was more effective in lowering the duration of migraines.

What the Research Tells Us

These studies demonstrate that 5-HTP can decrease migraine frequency and severity in many people. Indeed, in a comparison with propranolol, a first-line drug prescribed by thousands of doctors to treat this problem, 5-HTP demonstrated a statistically significant ability to reduce migraine attacks.

Because 5-HTP is natural to the body, it causes few side effects, which are almost always mild and can be lessened by lowering the dosage. They include sedation, unusual dreams, and, in a small number of users, gastric discomfort. On the other hand, the list of propranolol's potential side effects is long. Years ago, I had to take propranolol for a period of time. My gums receded and my ability to exercise decreased greatly. I hope never to take it again.

Interestingly, 5-HTP has also been proven to reduce childhood migraines. (See "Preventing Migraines in Children and Adolescents" on page 107.)

Dosage

The standard starting dosage of 5-HTP is 50 to 100 mg. The maximum dosage is approximately 300 to 400 mg. Higher dosages have been used, but you should work with an alternative doctor before raising your amount. Start with a low dosage and increase it gradually, if necessary. Check the label of the product you choose for specific dosage recommendations and limits. This supplement should be taken at bedtime.

NIACIN

Niacin, also called vitamin B_3 or nicotinic acid, is natural to the human body and essential for health. First identified in 1873, niacin has an average RDI of 15 mg. A deficiency in this vitamin leads to pellagra, a disease that is characterized by skin abnormalities, inflammation of the mouth, abdominal problems, delirium, and, if left untreated, death. Pellagra is rarely seen in advanced societies, and when it is seen, it is usually the result of alcoholism or drug abuse.

Niacin is best known medically for its ability to lower total cholesterol, low-density lipoproteins (LDL cholesterol), and triglycerides. Actually, niacin was the first therapy found to reduce total cholesterol and LDL levels. Additionally, niacin increases high-density lipoprotein (HDL cholesterol) levels, often called the "good cholesterol." In fact, it boosts HDL cholesterol far better than the pharmaceuticals typically prescribed to control cholesterol, including statin drugs. For these reasons, niacin is often recommended by both mainstream and alternative doctors to treat unhealthful cholesterol levels.

Despite the well-known uses of niacin, few mainstream or alternative practitioners know about this vitamin's ability to prevent and even halt migraine headaches.

How It Works

Because niacin is a potent vasodilator, some researchers have hypothesized that it works by opening the constricted cerebral blood vessels that precede migraine attacks. This explanation, however, does not seem plausible, because highly dilated cerebral blood vessels are thought to be the cause of migraine pain itself. In fact, many prescription and natural migraine remedies prevent migraines or halt acute attacks by blocking extreme blood vessel dilation and promoting vasoconstriction. Thus, if the hypothesis above is true, niacin would actually cause migraines. Indeed, one of niacin's common side effects is headaches, although not migraines.

One theory behind niacin's successful treatment of migraines is that it somehow alters the vasodilation that occurs in the arteries associated with migraines by causing a body-wide vasodilation, commonly known as a "niacin flush." This action, in turn, reduces or halts the pain produced by migraine vasodilation. Another explanation for niacin's effectiveness is that it increases plasma concentrations of serotonin by preventing tryptophan, a precursor of serotonin, from being shunted into other biochemical pathways. Thus, tryptophan is reliably converted to serotonin, which, in turn, causes vasoconstriction in the cerebral arteries in some people and reduces migraines. Another possibility is niacin's ability to enhance energy metabolism in mitochondria, which has been linked to effective migraine therapy.

Scientific Reports of Niacin's Effectiveness

As you can see, the mechanism by which niacin prevents or halts migraines in some people is not exactly known. Today, a statement made in 1949 by Dr. R. Grenfell in still stands: "Theoretically it is hard to see how a vasodilator [niacin] can stop an attack of migraine."[42] Yet, as the following evidence indicates, niacin actually can treat these headaches.

● **1944 (First Report).** In a study published in the *Annals of Internal Medicine,* Dr. Miles Atkinson treated twenty-one patients that were suffering from long-term migraines.[43] Using various combinations of intravenous, intramuscular, and oral niacin, seventeen patients (81 percent) reported substantial improvement. Two of these seventeen patients obtained complete remission, ten others gained great improvement, and another five saw moderate improvement. Of the eight people with frequent incapacitating headaches, five obtained great relief, while three experienced moderate relief.

Before obtaining great relief with the help of niacin treatment, one twenty-year-old woman averaged one incapacitating headache a week, which made it impossible for her to work. She also got two or three less severe migraines per week. With niacin therapy, however, she experienced only a mild migraine every two months.

In another case, a lawyer's migraines were so severe that he sometimes beat his head against a wall. He endured these migraines three times a month, in addition to many lesser migraine headaches. After nine months of niacin treatment, he no longer experienced any severe migraines, and had only a few minor ones. According to the author, the attorney would get a migraine after "some gross indiscretion of living [excessive drinking]." Still, the attorney kept his perspective, saying, "You can't reasonably expect this stuff [niacin] to prevent a hangover!"

Important to note is the fact that some of the study's subjects reported immediate relief from acute migraines as a result of the niacin injections. (See "Natural Remedies for Acute Migraines" on page 117.)

● **2003.** A sixty-two-year-old woman with a forty-year history of moderately severe migraines was seen as an outpatient at the Mayo Clinic in Arizona.[44] Her migraines lasted twenty-four to forty-eight hours and were accompanied by nausea and vomiting, as well as sensitivity to light, noise, and movement. She had previously taken prescription triptan drugs (injectable sumatriptan or oral zolmitriptan), which provided some relief. During the nine months prior to trying niacin, however, her migraines had become worse and more frequent, which she attributed to the loss of her son and moving across the country.

A friend told her that his migraines had ceased since he began taking niacin to treat his cholesterol problem. The woman started to take 750 mg of over-the-counter sustained-release niacin every day. This therapy of 375 mg of niacin twice a day stopped her migraines.

When the woman's doctor advised her that sustained-release niacin has been linked to liver injury, they agreed that she would reduce the dosage to 375 mg once daily. With this regimen, she experienced only two mild migraines over two months. Although the doctor was right about sustained-release niacin's potential to cause liver irritation, this side effect is infrequent, and the liver injury is reversible with the discontinuation of niacin. In addition, amounts of 375 mg of niacin once or twice daily are already low dosages.

Additional Evidence

In addition to the 1944 study mentioned earlier, four other reports that show niacin's ability to halt acute migraine attacks can be found in "Natural Remedies for Acute Migraines" on page 117.

What the Research Tells Us

As the studies prove, niacin can reduce the frequency of migraines and even stop acute migraine attacks. In emergency rooms, however, doctors treat acute, severe migraines with triptan drugs and major painkillers, all of which can have serious side effects. In doctors' offices, migraine sufferers are prescribed drugs that also have many risks. Niacin, like riboflavin, can be used for acute or chronic migraines. In fact, the evidence of its ability to treat acute migraines is particularly strong. In the same way that emergency room doctors should consider using oral or intravenous magnesium to treat acute migraines (see "Magnesium" on page 35), they should also try oral or intravenous niacin before turning to injectable triptan drugs, which have caused cardiovascular complications that include heart attacks and death.

Plain niacin is the fastest acting form of this supplement, and in one case report, acute migraine attacks were halted with dosages of 300 to 500 mg. Niacin therapy, however, may come with side effects. It can cause intense flushing and itching of the skin that some people find very unpleasant. In one of the studies described earlier, about 15 percent of subjects found the "niacin flush" more unpleasant than the migraine itself. Yet, the other subjects found niacin to be worth taking to prevent or halt their migraines.

Sometimes the flushing caused by plain niacin may be reduced with over-the-counter aspirin, ibuprofen (Motrin), or naproxen (Aleve). It is not known whether a decrease in the flushing would lower niacin's effectiveness in halting or preventing migraines.

Another way to reduce this side effect is to use sustained-release niacin. In the case reported from the Mayo Clinic, sustained-release niacin, which is available over-the-counter, was highly effective in preventing migraines in a woman who had been suffering from frequent migraines for many years. Sustained-release niacin is absorbed slowly into the body, therefore reducing the tendency for flushing. Nevertheless, some flushing may still occur. If you try sustained-release niacin, start with the lowest dosage, increasing it slowly if you do not notice any benefits. Many mainstream doctors have considerable experience using niacin for patients with high cholesterol, so they should be able to help you in the use of this supplement for migraines.

Many alternative doctors have experience with a niacin supplement known as "no-flush niacin." Chemically, it is known as inositol hexaniacinate, or simply hexanicotinate. No-flush niacin does not contain niacin itself, but instead a molecule consisting of inositol and a ring of niacin esters. It causes very little flushing. There is some debate about whether or not no-flush niacin works, but I have personally seen it increase the HDL cholesterol (good cholesterol) and lower the LDL cholesterol (bad cholesterol). Its effect on migraines, however, is not known.

Dosage

Whichever form of niacin you choose, I recommend working with your health care practitioner. Niacin preparations can affect blood glucose, uric acid, cholesterol, and liver enzyme levels, so these should be checked after a few months of niacin treatment.

If you use oral niacin, start with a low dosage of 50 or 100 mg a day, which is the best way to minimize the flushing, nausea, itching, or other adverse effects that may occur with this therapy. Compounding pharmacies can fashion niacin pills of any size to fit your individual tolerance. Increase your dosage gradually, if needed. If you use no-flush niacin, start with the lowest dose, which is usually 500 mg.

VITAMIN D

Also known as calciferol, vitamin D is best recognized for its essential role in the maintenance of healthy bones, which it performs along with calcium and other minerals. Vitamin D comprises a number of different forms, including vitamin D_2 and D_3, which act more like hormones than vitamins in the human body. The vitamin D_3 type is produced in humans when skin is exposed to ultraviolet light from the sun.

Recent studies suggest that vitamin D deficiency affects one third of adults. This is an important finding because low levels of this substance have been associated with high blood pressure, diabetes, stroke, heart attack, kidney disease, immune system impairment, fibromyalgia, osteoporosis, and a dozen types of cancer, including breast, colon, and prostate cancers. Vitamin D also produces hormones that regulate hundreds of genes. In fact, scientific inquiry suggests that a vitamin D deficiency affects almost every system of the body.

Uncertainty remains over what blood level constitutes a vitamin D deficiency. In general, an amount of 30 to 40 ng/ml (nanograms per milliliter) is considered adequate, although an increasing number of experts believe that a higher level is optimal, and that anything less represents a vitamin D deficiency. In terms of treating migraine headaches, the cases reported below suggest that higher blood levels of vitamin D may be required to properly treat this problem.

How It Works

Unfortunately, the relationship of vitamin D and migraine headaches is not understood at this time. There is, nevertheless, abundant evidence of vitamin D's ability to prevent migraines, as the following reports show.

Scientific Reports of Vitamin D's Effectiveness

Although the evidence presented in this chapter is limited, these cases provide migraineurs a reason to have their vitamin D levels tested and, if necessary, corrected.

● **1994 (First Report).** In the first peer-reviewed cases of vitamin D's role in migraine treatment, Dr. Susan Thys-Jacobs described "dramatic reduction" in severe migraines with the use of vitamin D_3 and calcium in two female subjects.[45] The first woman was fifty years old and had a five-year history of excruciating migraines. Symptoms included brief bilateral blindness, and numbness and tingling in her right arm. She endured two to three migraines a week, each of which lasted four hours to a few days. Prescription drugs were not helpful. The woman's vitamin D_3 level of 19.8 ng/ml was considered low-normal in 1994, but today, it would be deemed low.

Treatment with 50,000 IU weekly of vitamin D_3 along with 1,000 mg daily of calcium reduced migraine attacks from eight to one per month. Maintaining the woman's vitamin D_3 level over 40 ng/ml greatly decreased the frequency and duration of her migraines.

According to another case listed in the report, a sixty-five-year-old woman had been experiencing occasional migraines for forty years. When she was sixty-three, she had a stroke and subsequent neurosurgery, and ever since experienced three to four excruciating migraines per week. Her vitamin D_3 level was low at 15 ng/ml. Therapy with vitamin D_3 at

50,000 IU per week and calcium at 2,000 mg per day produced "a dramatic reduction" in migraine attacks, cutting them to approximately one per month. A subsequent vitamin D_3 level was 52 ng/ml.

That same year, Dr. Susan Thys-Jacobs published another article regarding the benefits of vitamin D and calcium.[46] It described two women who had experienced severe migraines for over twenty-five years. The worst migraines occurred during the premenstrual phases of their menstrual cycles. Treatment with standard medications provided little benefit, yet a combination of vitamin D and calcium produced substantial improvement.

● **2008.** In a review of records that covered a six-month period in 2007 at a headache center in Florida, fifty-four patients, forty of whom were women, were identified with chronic migraines.[47] The average age of the subjects was fifty, ranging from seventeen to seventy-three. Twenty-two subjects (41 percent) had low vitamin D levels, and only 7 percent of them were receiving adequate vitamin D supplementation. Unfortunately, this study did not take the next step, which would be to prescribe vitamin D supplementation to those with vitamin D deficiency. Yet, the association of low vitamin D levels and migraines in this survey does suggest that a substantial number of people with migraines may be deficient in vitamin D. This may, in turn, explain the good results obtained by Dr. Thys-Jacobs in the previously mentioned studies.

● **2009.** In 2009, Dr. Sanjay Prakash and colleagues published an article discussing vitamin D deficiencies in people with chronic headaches. This article reported the effectiveness of vitamin D therapy in people with chronic tension headaches and vitamin D deficiencies.[48]

● **2010.** A second article by Dr. Prakash and colleagues reviewed the available literature and found a significant correlation between both tension headaches and migraines and latitude.[49] Headache prevalence increased at higher latitudes, as well as with the autumn and winter seasons. Having shown that chronic tension headaches responded to vitamin D only a year earlier, the authors connected these findings by suggesting that the higher occurrence of tension and migraine headaches at increased latitudes (that is, closer to the poles) might be directly related to low vitamin D levels.

Of course, insufficient vitamin D levels are expected at higher latitudes, where the intensity of sunlight, especially in autumn and winter, is low. For example, both the duration and intensity of sunlight are more limited in Boston, which sits at a relatively high latitude on the globe, than they are in Miami, which sits at a low latitude. Perhaps the greater occurrence of migraine and tension headaches in northern climates is due in part to vitamin D deficiencies. The improvements experienced by Dr. Prakash's patients of 2009 suggest this may be correct.

Additional Evidence

The following testimonial was posted in the newspaper columns section of the online health resource The People's Pharmacy:

I started taking vitamin D_3 supplements about a year ago when my doctor tested my blood and found out I was vitamin D deficient. Is it just a coincidence that my migraines and chronic headaches have almost disappeared? I've had them for over 25 years and I am glad not to be suffering.[50]

People with twenty-five-year histories of migraines have usually tried everything mainstream medicine offers, including prescription and over-the-counter drugs, and even some supplements. If nothing has worked, it is obvious that these people are not susceptible to placebo cures. When a new therapy—in this case, vitamin D—provides a major reduction in headache frequency that lasts more than six months, it is significant. My feeling is that a collection of reports such as this one is as valuable as any large double-blind, placebo-controlled study.

What the Research Tells Us

Major medical problems can develop in long-term migraine sufferers and also in people with long-term vitamin D deficiencies. If your vitamin D level is low, supplementation with this vitamin should be considered first as a treatment for your migraines. It is the easiest method to try. The fact that medical science does not yet understand vitamin D's role in migraine therapy does not mean you won't get good results from using this vitamin.

Dosage

Mainstream medical institutions now recommend vitamin D dosages of 200 to 800 IU per day to maintain adequate vitamin D levels. Other mainstream and alternative experts, however, treat patients with 2,000 to 5,000 IU per day, and sometimes more. Also note that 1,000 mg per day of calcium was used in some of the successful cases noted earlier.

If you are using these higher doses of vitamin D, it is essential that you see your doctor to obtain vitamin D blood levels. Vitamin D toxicity can occur, causing weakness, constipation, nausea, and heart rhythm irregularity. Excessive vitamin D or calcium may also cause calcium deposits in the arteries. I advise working with your health care practitioner to monitor your blood regularly until your vitamin D level is optimal.

3. HERBAL REMEDIES

As their name suggests, herbal remedies are medicinal substances extracted from plants. Herbal therapy has long been an integral part of modern medicine. In fact, approximately 25 percent of modern prescription drugs were originally derived from plants. Plant-based medicine has been used to treat a number of health conditions over the years. For example, digitalis, a standard treatment for heart failure for more than a century, is derived from the flowering plant foxglove. Another herb, colchicine, is still used to relieve gout and Mediterranean fever. In addition, several herbal remedies have been proven to provide significant benefits in the treatment of migraines in both adults and children.

FEVERFEW

For centuries, herbalists have used the plant feverfew (*Tanacetum parthenium*) to treat fever, rheumatism, toothache, stomach ache, insect bites, asthma, and headache. Since the middle of the twentieth century, it has also been used to prevent migraines.

How It Works

As stated earlier, serotonin plays a major role in the development of migraines. The most popular pre-

scription drugs for halting acute migraines are trip-
tans, which impact serotonin receptors in the blood
vessels of the brain. Yet triptan drugs have too many
risks to be taken daily as a migraine treatment. Feverfew also impacts the serotonin system, blocking serotonin receptors 5-HT2A and 5-HT2C. In doing so, it can
also prevent migraines.[1,2] Additionally, feverfew
reduces inflammation by inhibiting the synthesis of
prostaglandins, the hormone-like substances that mod-
ulate inflammation, thereby helping to reduce pain.

Scientific Reports of Feverfew's Effectiveness

The research that has been conducted over the past
few decades builds a strong case for feverfew's use as
migraine therapy. As the following reports show,
treatment with this herb produces less and milder side
effects than the pharmaceuticals used to prevent
migraines, making it well worth consideration.

• **1985 (First Report).** In the August 1985 issue of the
British Medical Journal, Dr. E. Johnson and colleagues
reported the results of a double-blind, placebo-controlled study that used feverfew to prevent migraine
headaches.[3] Of the eight subjects that received feverfew, seven demonstrated a marked reduction in
migraine frequency. This group averaged 7.5 migraines
in the month prior to therapy, yet suffered only 1.5
migraines per month after six months of feverfew
treatment—an average decrease of 80 percent.

Many of the individual results were remarkable.
For example, subject 1 experienced twelve migraine

attacks during the baseline month, yet had no migraines during the final three months of feverfew therapy. Subject 6 suffered eight to twelve migraines per month during baseline, yet experienced only two migraines during the final three months—in other words, less than one attack per month with feverfew treatment. Subject 2 averaged eight migraine attacks per month during baseline, but had only one migraine per month while taking feverfew.

Whereas seven of the eight subjects that received feverfew experienced substantial decreases in migraine frequency, only one of the nine subjects in the placebo group saw any reduction in migraine frequency—and a very slight one at that.

Subjects in the feverfew group reported five minor side effects, including joint stiffness, palpitations, abdominal pain, mouth ulcer, and heavy menstruation. The placebo subjects listed nineteen. No serious side effects occurred in either group.

● **1988.** In this double-blind, placebo-controlled, crossover study, feverfew proved superior to placebo according to several aspects of migraine prevention.[4] Among the fifty-nine subjects, the average number of migraine attacks was 4.7 over two months of placebo therapy. In contrast, the feverfew group averaged 3.6 migraines, which represented a 24-percent drop in migraines. In addition, the headaches were milder with feverfew therapy, which also yielded a significant reduction in the accompanying nausea and vomiting.

Side effects occurred more frequently in the placebo group. The most common adverse reactions with feverfew were mouth ulceration, indigestion, heartburn, and lightheadedness. No serious side effects were reported.

● **1997.** Forty-seven women and ten men, averaging thirty-eight years old (ranging from nine to sixty-five), were involved in this double-blind, placebo-controlled study of feverfew.[5] Many of these patients (43 percent) sustained more than ten migraine attacks per month. None had taken feverfew previously.

The primary measurement of effectiveness was a reduction in migraine pain intensity. In all three phases of the study, feverfew significantly lowered pain intensity in comparison with the placebo. Using a pain scale of 2 (very mild) to 10 (severe), therapy with feverfew decreased subjects' pain intensity from an average of 9.5 to 3 over four months. In comparison, when subjects received the placebo, pain intensity increased. Feverfew also significantly lessened the subjects' symptoms of vomiting and sensitivity to light.

The researchers commented, "The results show clearly that feverfew brought about a significant reduction in the intensity of migraine attacks."[6]

● **2002.** In this sixteen-week randomized, double-blind, placebo-controlled study, 147 migraine patients were treated with three different strengths of feverfew or a placebo.[7] In the groups that received the placebo or a very mild dosage of feverfew, scant reduction in migraine frequency was seen. In the group that took a moderate dosage of feverfew, average migraine frequency was reduced from 4.8 migraines per month before treatment to 3 migraines per month with treatment, an improvement of approximately 35 percent. In the group that was given a high dosage of feverfew, migraine frequency decreased about 30 percent.

Nearly one-third of subjects in the moderate-dosage and high-dosage groups obtained a 50-percent reduction in migraine occurrence. Fifty-three percent of subjects that took a moderate dosage of feverfew reported a good or very good response.

Side effects occurred equally with feverfew and placebo, and there were no serious adverse reactions.

● **2005.** In a European study involving people with long histories of migraines, eighty-nine subjects received 6.25 mg of feverfew three times a day for sixteen weeks.[8] Eighty-one subjects received a placebo for the same period of time. The average age of the subjects was forty-three, 83 percent of them were female, and each experienced approximately five migraine attacks per month.

Migraine frequency was reduced on average from 4.8 attacks per month prior to feverfew treatment to 2.9 attacks per month with this therapy—a decrease of nearly 40 percent. Thirty percent of patients in the feverfew group experienced a 50-percent or greater reduction in migraine occurrence. The average number of days per month that subjects had migraines was 7 before feverfew treatment and approximately 4.5 after—a reduction of nearly 40 percent. Migraine duration was also lowered. Much smaller decreases in these measurements were seen with placebo treatment.

In overall effectiveness, feverfew therapy was statistically superior to treatment with a placebo. Moreover, the doctors conducting the study rated 54 percent of feverfew users as having a good or very good response. In addition, the majority of subjects taking feverfew rated themselves as having a good or very good response.

The tolerability of feverfew was high, equaling the tolerability of the placebo. Side effects were mostly mild and occurred in a similar number of feverfew and placebo patients.

Additional Evidence

Further proof of feverfew's ability to prevent migraines can be found at the online resource The People's Pharmacy, where one reader stated:

> I started taking feverfew for migraine headaches in 1998 and haven't had a migraine since then.[9]

Additionally, evidence of feverfew's effectiveness comes indirectly from the drug industry. Specifically, the drugs cyproheptadine (Periactin) and pizotifen (Sandomigran, which is not available in the United States) have proven to prevent migraines by blocking the same serotonin receptors (5-HT2A and 5-HT2C) that feverfew blocks. Also, from personal experience, I can say that feverfew, like cyproheptadine and pizotifen, causes constriction of the small arteries, which can prevent migraines.

What the Research Tells Us

The reports of feverfew's ability to treat migraines are convincing. The available information shows that feverfew can be highly effective in reducing the frequency, intensity, and duration of migraine headaches. For some people, feverfew can be as or more powerful than prescription drugs. Its side effects are fewer and milder than those of pharmaceuticals and disappear with discontinuance of treatment.

Dosage

Because different manufacturers produce feverfew in different concentrations, I cannot recommend a specific dosage. Simply purchase feverfew that is made by a reputable manufacturer and follow the directions on the label. The quality of natural supplements is likely to be higher at a health food store than in catalogues that advertise low-cost options.

Information on feverfew's use during pregnancy is scant. Women who are pregnant or breastfeeding, or who are planning to become pregnant, should speak to their doctors before taking feverfew. In some people, feverfew may slow blood clotting. If you are taking any substance that inhibits blood clotting, such as warfarin (Coumadin), aspirin, clopidogrel (Plavix), fish oils, or nattokinase, ask your doctor before starting feverfew therapy. Feverfew can interact with many prescription drugs, so if you are taking any medication, talk to your doctor or pharmacist.

Feverfew should not be discontinued abruptly if you have benefited from its use. Stopping cold turkey may lead to a rebound of migraines. If you have obtained only partial improvement after trying fever-few, you may want to consider the two prescription drugs mentioned earlier (cyproheptadine and pizo-tifen), which work similarly to feverfew and may pro-vide you with better results. (While pizotifen is not available in the United States, it is accessible in Canada.) As previously noted, both drugs are serotonin antagonists that block serotonin receptors 5-HT2A and 5-HT2C, just like feverfew does. If you'd prefer to avoid pharmaceuticals, the herb white willow also has similar properties, and can be combined with feverfew for increased effectiveness in migraine prevention.

WHITE WILLOW

The Chinese, Greeks, and Romans have used white willow as an herbal remedy for thousands of years to relieve fever and pain. It is obtained from the bark of the white willow tree (Salix alba), which is indigenous to Europe and Asia. One of the most important histor-ical reports of white willow was recorded in 1763 when Edward Stone described its positive effect in the treatment of malaria.[10]

Identified in the 1800s, the active ingredient in white willow is called salacin.[11,12] By the early twenti-eth century, a pure form of salacin from white willow was marketed. Soon thereafter it was synthesized as aspirin (acetylsalicylic acid), the world's most used drug. Aspirin is more potent than salacin, but it is also more prone to causing side effects such as stomach irritation, ulcers, and internal bleeding. Salacin is much gentler on the stomach than aspirin.[13,14]

White willow is often recommended by herbalists for the treatment of sore throat, joint discomfort and pain, backache, menstrual pain, toothache, and fever and muscle aches caused by colds or the flu. Several studies show that white willow can even be an effective therapy for osteoarthritis.[15] It also has antioxidant properties.

How It Works

As previously explained, migraine headaches can be prevented by substances that block the serotonin receptors 5-HT2A and 5-HT2C in the arteries of the brain. Like feverfew, white willow impedes these receptors and can inhibit migraines.

Scientific Reports of White Willow's Effectiveness

Despite the strong theoretical basis for white willow's effectiveness in the treatment of migraines, as yet there are no studies regarding the use of this plant alone to prevent these headaches. Fortunately, there is one study of white willow's use along with feverfew, and it is compelling enough to include white willow on the list of natural migraine remedies.

● **2006 (First Report).** Conducted in France, this study involved seven women and five men of an average age of thirty-six, ranging from eighteen to fifty years old.[16] The subjects' history of migraines varied from six months to thirty-six years. Headache frequency ranged from one every two weeks to three per week. Each subject received 300 mg of white willow and 300 mg of feverfew twice daily.

The primary factor measured by this study was migraine frequency. After six weeks of white willow-feverfew treatment, migraine frequency was reduced by 57 percent on average. Over the following six weeks, average migraine frequency dropped even further, falling 62 percent on average. In fact, 90 percent of subjects experienced a substantial reduction in migraine frequency. This is an excellent result, and a far better one than those of most migraines drugs.

The white willow-feverfew combination also markedly lowered migraine pain intensity, which decreased by an average of 39 percent after six weeks of the herbal therapy. After three months, it fell 63 percent on average. Every subject experienced a reduction in migraine pain intensity.

When the study began, the average duration of a migraine attack was thirty-three hours. After six weeks of white willow-feverfew treatment, the average duration was eleven hours—a 67-percent improvement. At the end of the study, the average migraine duration had dropped even further to eight hours—a 72-percent reduction. Migraine attack duration was reduced in all subjects. By the study's end, significant improvements were also seen in the subjects' quality of life measurements. No notable side effects with white willow-feverfew treatment were reported.

The doctors concluded, "In the current study, the combination of [feverfew and white willow] was remarkably effective in reducing attack frequency, pain intensity and duration." Although doctors are known to overstate their results at times, this doctor's conclusion was no exaggeration.

What the Research Tells Us

The results of the research on white willow and fever-few as combination migraine therapy are highly impressive in comparison with other natural remedies or frequently used pharmaceuticals. So, although this white willow-feverfew study is small and the only one of its kind, its findings deserve attention. Further study of white willow is badly needed, but that will take years to accomplish. In the meantime, the combination of feverfew and white willow is worth considering among the natural therapies for migraine headaches. It is certainly a good option to try before you take prescription drugs.

Dosage

In the recently described study, a product called Mig-RL was used. Unfortunately, I was not able to find Mig-RL for purchase anywhere. An online search using the terms "white willow feverfew" reveals many products by various companies, but choosing one can be challenging, as various brands offer different concentrations or dosages of the two herbs. The best approach is simply to follow dosage guidelines of the product you purchase. There is one product called MigraDefense that contains not only feverfew and white willow but also magnesium and butterbur. My recommendation is to try either feverfew or white willow on its own first before taking a combination supplement. You may need only one of these remedies, not both.

If you are allergic to aspirin, you should not take white willow. White willow should not be used in youths under the age of eighteen who have the flu or other viral conditions because of the potential for serious medical complications, particularly Reye's syndrome. White willow has a mild anticoagulant effect, so talk to your doctor before using this therapy if you are taking aspirin, warfarin (Coumadin), omega-3 fatty acids (fish oils), nattokinase, or other blood-thinning substances. Also, do not take white willow with anti-inflammatory medication such as ibuprofen or naproxen. Always check with your doctor about mixing white willow with prescription medications.

As previously mentioned, there are two prescription drugs that work similarly to white willow and feverfew in the prevention of migraines: cyproheptadine (Periactin) and pizotifen (Sandomigran). Both are serotonin antagonists and, like feverfew and white willow, block receptors 5-HT2A and 5-HT2C. If these herbal therapies do not provide adequate relief, one of these medications might. Pizotifen, however, is not available in the United States, but may be ordered from Canada.

BUTTERBUR

Butterbur (*Petasites hybridus*) has been used as a folk medicine for over two thousand years. It is a perennial shrub that is native to North America, Europe, and Southeastern Asia, and is usually found along rivers and streams, and in damp forests and marshy areas.

Since the middle of the twentieth century, western science has taken an interest in butterbur as a remedy for cough, seasonal allergies, asthma, and allergic skin conditions. The usage of butterbur that has displayed the most promise, however, is in the prevention of migraine headaches. Although butterbur has proven medicinal properties, it is considered a natural product in the United States and the United Kingdom, and is available as an herbal supplement. In Germany, however, butterbur requires a doctor's prescription.

How It Works

The mechanism by which butterbur extract reduces migraine attacks is not precisely known. The medically active substances in butterbur include petasin and isopetasin. These natural chemical compounds are believed to have calcium-blocking properties similar to magnesium and drugs such as diltiazem (Cardizem) and amlodipine (Norvasc), all of which are used to prevent migraines. These treatments work by reducing spasms in the small arteries of the body and brain. Another possibility is that butterbur may have anti-inflammatory effects that inhibit leukotrienes, which are inflammatory substances potentially involved in the development of migraines.

Scientific Reports of Butterbur's Effectiveness

Although Native Americans have used butterbur for centuries to alleviate headache and inflammation, this natural therapy has only recently undergone scientific study. Nevertheless, the research that has been released proves the herb to be a truly promising method of migraine prevention.

● **2000 (First Report).** Fifty-nine people with a history of chronic migraines were included in a randomized, placebo-controlled, double-blind study of butterbur extract. The subjects' ages ranged from eighteen to sixty, and thirty-two of the participants were female. After four weeks without any migraine therapy, a twelve-week period began, during which thirty-two of the subjects received 25 mg of butterbur extract twice a day, while twenty-seven patients received a placebo.

The study focused primarily on butterbur's ability to reduce the frequency of migraine attacks. During the month without treatment, the subjects in the butterbur extract group experienced 3.4 migraines on average. By the third month of butterbur therapy, that number dropped to 1.8—a reduction of approximately 47 percent. Some subjects achieved 60-percent decreases in migraine frequency. Considering the low dosage used in this study, this was a very good result. In comparison, subjects who received the placebo saw much less improvement. Their average monthly migraine frequency fell from 2.9 to 2.6—a decrease of only 10 percent.

Treatment Group	Migraine Frequency Without Treatment	Migraine Frequency After Third Month of Treatment	Improvement
Butterbur	3.4	1.8	47%
Placebo	2.9	2.6	10%

The improvement with butterbur was statistically significant in comparison to placebo. The authors concluded, "The combination of high efficacy and excellent tolerance emphasizes the particular value that Petasites hybridus has for the prophylactic treatment of migraine." Although this study was conducted between 1993 and 1995, it was not reported until 2000.[17] An analysis of even greater depth was published in 2004.[18]

● **2004.** Larger doses than the amount administered in the 2000 study were investigated in this randomized, double-blind clinical trial of butterbur extract.[19] A total of 202 chronic migraine sufferers took part, ranging from age eighteen to sixty-five, and 82 percent were female. Prior to this research, they experienced two to seven migraine attacks per month.

The study consisted of three groups. One group received 75 mg of butterbur extract twice a day, one group took 50 mg of butterbur extract twice a day, and the third was given a placebo. Over four months of treatment, migraine occurrence dropped an average of 45 percent in the group receiving 75 mg of butterbur twice daily. This result was statistically significant. Sixty-eight percent of the subjects in this group obtained a 50-percent or greater reduction in migraine frequency. These results equaled or exceeded those associated with many migraine medications. Over the same time frame, those taking 50 mg of butterbur extract twice daily averaged a 32-percent decrease in migraine occurrence. Clearly, the larger dosage of butterbur was more effective.

The effectiveness of butterbur increased toward the end of the study. This is not unusual with natural remedies, which seem to require three to six months to reach maximum impact. Indeed, even better results may have been seen had butterbur been given for six instead of three months.

Adverse effects were reported almost equally between the butterbur and placebo groups. The only side effects seen more commonly with butterbur than placebo were stomach problems (mostly burping).

The doctors conducting this study concluded, "The results from this study support the efficacy of Petasites extract (butterbur) as a preventive therapy for migraine. . . . The magnitude of the treatment effect for the 75 mg dose of Petasites was substantial. . . . This level of treatment effect is broadly comparable with results obtained with prescription preventive medications."

● **2005.** A total of 108 children and adolescents with a year or more of repeated migraine headaches participated in this study, which used 50 to 150 mg of butterbur extract per day, depending on the subject's age.[20] Seventy-seven percent of butterbur recipients reported a reduction in migraine frequency of 50 percent or greater—an excellent response. (For a detailed description of this study, see "Preventing Migraines in Children and Adolescents" on page 107.)

What the Research Tells Us

The research on butterbur makes a convincing case for this herbal remedy's ability to prevent migraines. In fact, some experts believe butterbur to be the most effective and reliable herb for treating migraines.

The studies listed above were conducted with a brand name product of butterbur called Petadolex.

This supplement is a refined extract of the herb. It is important to use a refined extract rather than a whole plant product, as unrefined butterbur contains substances that may cause liver injury or cancer. These substances are removed in the production of most butterbur extracts marketed by reliable companies today.

Dosage

The dosage of butterbur extract is usually 50 or 75 mg twice a day. Infrequent side effects with butterbur include stomach pain, nausea, and burping.

GINGER

For centuries, herbalists in Europe and Asia have used ginger to treat common conditions such as nausea, gastric pain, vomiting, tension headaches, and migraines. Derived from the plant *Zingiber officinale*, ginger has received considerable study as a treatment for the nausea and vomiting that can accompany pregnancy and chemotherapy.

How It Works

Little is known about how ginger might help prevent migraines. Ginger has anti-inflammatory, antihistamine, antibacterial, and antioxidant effects, but how these or ginger's other medicinal properties might inhibit migraines is not known.

Scientific Reports of Ginger's Effectiveness

Although research on ginger's ability to prevent migraines is limited, case reports like the following warrant serious consideration and suggest that ginger may be an option if more popular therapies fail.

● **1990 (First Report).** As described in a case report published in the *Journal of Ethnopharmacology*, a forty-two-year-old woman obtained substantial relief from her migraines by using ginger.[21] At twenty-six, the woman began to suffer from mild migraines, which increased in frequency and severity over the next fifteen years. At this point, she was prescribed the ergot medication dihydroergotamine (DHE). The drug worked well, but because of potentially serious adverse effects, the woman stopped taking it. After two months, her migraines gradually returned. At the onset of another migraine, her doctors gave her approximately 500 to 600 mg of powdered ginger in water, and her migraine abated within minutes. She continued using this remedy a couple of times each day for several days, and her migraine did not return.

Because of her excellent response, the woman began adding uncooked ginger to her daily diet. This produced a marked reduction in migraine occurrence. In the following thirteen months, she had only six migraines of mild intensity.

The doctors commented, "We propose that consumption of powdered or fresh ginger should exert abortive and prophylactic effects in migraine headache. . . . No side effects of ginger root consumption have been documented. Therefore, it could be also useful in childhood and juvenile migraine."

● **2005.** Homeopathic treatment is based on the theory that tiny amounts of a medicinal substance can have a major impact on the human system. This explanation has never made sense to me scientifically, but now and then I meet people who say that homeopathic remedies work for them. Homeopathy is usually very safe, so there is little risk in trying it.

Purported to reduce or stop acute migraines, the homeopathic remedy known as GelStat was evaluated in a 2005 open-label study of migraine sufferers. Containing trace amounts of ginger and feverfew, GelStat proved to be an effective treatment. In addition, GelStat lists many testimonials of its product's effectiveness on its website:

> I have tried every product available for my migraines. Nothing works. Even prescription medications from my doctor didn't help. I'm tired of using Advil and Motrin. I finally found the answer to my problem—GelStat.[22]

Further discussion of this remedy can be found in "Natural Remedies for Acute Migraines" on page 117.

Additional Evidence

In 2008, health website The People's Pharmacy posted the following letter from a reader regarding ginger's beneficial effect on migraines.

> Someone was asking about natural migraine remedies and you mentioned spicy hot and sour soup, among other things. I've had migraines since before I was in kindergarten (I'm 58 now), and the best thing I've found is ginger. Jamaican-style ginger beer (stronger than ginger ale) is good, though rather sweet. The pickled ginger sold with sushi is a godsend. It also helps with the nausea.[23]

As you know, anecdotal data can sometimes be just as helpful as reports from large studies. This letter makes a good case for ginger's effectiveness in migraine treatment. If you try ginger and find that it works for your situation, then that is all the proof you need.

What the Research Tells Us

The scientific evidence for ginger's use in the prevention of migraines is limited. Furthermore, the findings on GelStat's ability to treat acute and chronic migraines are complicated by the fact that this product contains both ginger and feverfew, which raises the possibility of feverfew, not ginger, being the active ingredient. Even so, if GelStat works for you, isn't that the goal? And as the other cases above suggest, using ginger alone as a food or supplement may also be worth the attempt.

Dosage

Ginger can be purchased as a supplement, or you can use sliced ginger or the ginger drinks mentioned earlier. The usual daily dosage is 1 to 4 g. Start with the lowest dose and increase gradually if necessary.

Although ginger can cause side effects, it does not usually do so. The most common adverse reactions are stomach upset, heartburn, gas, and bloating. Ginger may also inhibit platelet aggregation, which means it can cause bleeding in people who have bleeding tendencies, or in those who take aspirin, fish oil, warfarin (Coumadin), or similar antiplatelet substances. Be sure to check with your doctor.

GINKGO BILOBA

Used by herbalists for thousands of years, ginkgo biloba is one of the best-selling herbal supplements in the United States. Derived from the dried green leaves of the ginkgo biloba tree, this extract is most commonly recommended to treat blood disorders and enhance memory, but may also reduce the occurrence of migraine headaches.

How It Works

Containing the chemically active compound called ginkgolide B, ginkgo biloba extract produces a potent anti-inflammatory effect by inhibiting a biological agent known as platelet activating factor (PAF). This agent causes inflammation when released by platelets and white blood cells. Additionally, ginkgo regulates the activity of the excitatory amino acid glutamine in the central nervous system. Finally, ginkgo is also a mild vasodilator that can be used as a complementary therapy in the treatment of high blood pressure, peripheral vascular disease, impaired blood flow from atherosclerosis, and neurological disorders such as dementia and Alzheimer's disease—and to prevent migraines.

Scientific Reports of Ginkgo Biloba's Effectiveness

Although limited in number, the studies on this subject thus far suggest that gingko may be a promising alternative to commonly prescribed migraine medications.

● **2009 (First Report).** A study of fifty women, each with a long-term migraine disorder, examined the ability of ginkgo biloba to inhibit migraines.[24] After a two-month baseline phase without any treatment, the women were treated twice daily over four months with a product called Migrasoll, which contains 60 mg of ginkgo biloba, 11 mg of coenzyme Q_{10}, and 8.7 mg of riboflavin. (The amounts of coenzyme Q_{10} and riboflavin in this product are tiny, so ginkgo was very likely the active ingredient.)

Migraine occurrence decreased from 3.7 per month at baseline to 2 per month after four months of treatment with ginkgo—a statistically significant reduction of 46 percent. Migraine duration also fell from forty minutes on average during baseline to eighteen minutes in the fourth month of treatment—a notable drop of 55 percent. By the fourth month of therapy, 42 percent of subjects were migraine free—an excellent result that far exceeds the effectiveness of most migraine drugs.

Migrasoll is available in Europe, but I cannot find it online, so it may not be available in North America. No Matter. You can simply purchase ginkgo itself at the same dosage found in Migrasoll (60 mg) and take it twice a day. Ginkgo can also be purchased at a higher dosage of 120 mg and taken twice a day if the lower dose is insufficient.

• **2010.** Twenty-four migraine sufferers between the ages of eight and eighteen were treated twice a day with a combination product that contained 80 mg of ginkgo, 20 mg of coenzyme Q_{10}, 1.6 mg of vitamin B_2 (riboflavin), and 300 mg of magnesium. A preliminary report in 2010 showed excellent results, and a final report in 2011 confirmed the effectiveness of this treatment.[25,26] (For further details on this study, see "Preventing Migraines in Children and Adolescents" on page 107.)

What the Research Tells Us

Based on the available research, ginkgo appears to be effective in significantly reducing migraine frequency and duration in the majority of users.

Dosage

Guidelines for gingko dosage are a bit complicated due to the varied concentrations of ginkgo biloba extract found in different manufacturers' products. The most common supplements contain 24 percent flavone glycosides, and recommend dosages of 40, 60, or 120 mg twice a day.

Infrequent side effects include headache, nausea, and stomach upset. In some people, ginkgo biloba can increase bleeding tendencies, so if you are taking any medication or supplement that diminishes blood clotting, such as aspirin, warfarin (Coumadin), or fish oil, or have a bleeding disorder, check with your doctor before trying ginkgo. If you are taking prescription medication, ask your pharmacist about possible interactions with this herbal supplement.

GAMMA LINOLENIC ACID

Although you might not think of oil as an herb, gamma linolenic acid (GLA) is an omega-6 fatty acid that is found in oils derived from herbal plants such as evening primrose, blackcurrant, and borage. GLA has traditionally been used to treat eczema, depression, chronic fatigue syndrome, muscle aches, menopausal hot flashes, premenstrual syndrome, and diabetic neuropathy. Its usefulness in the prevention of migraines, however, is not well known among health care professionals or the public.

How It Works

GLA causes the body to increase production of prostaglandin E1 (PGE1), which has anti-inflammatory effects that may reduce the inflammation associated with migraines. Through its effects on blood vessels, prostaglandin E1 may also reduce the vascular abnormalities associated with migraines.

Scientific Reports of GLA's Effectiveness

GLA's known biological effects suggest that this fatty acid may be a useful tool in the inhibition of migraines. The results of the following studies support this idea.

● **1997 (First Report).** A combination supplement containing 1800 mg of GLA and alpha linolenic acid (ALA), which also reduces inflammation, was studied for six months in 129 patients who suffered from long-term migraine disorders.[27] In addition to these oils, vitamin B_6 (pyridoxine), niacin, vitamin C, carotene, and vitamin E were also taken on a daily basis. The trial was open-label, meaning that the doctors and patients knew the nature of the treatment. The study did not have a placebo group, which weakens the certainty of the results, yet its benefits were so strong that they must be noted.

Improvement was not seen until the fourth month of therapy, and the best results occurred during the sixth and final month. Substantial benefits were gained by 86 percent of subjects, while only 14 percent experienced few or no positive results. Among those who achieved improvement, pain scale measurements dropped from 88 to 24 on average—a 73-percent reduction. In this group, migraine frequency fell by an average of nearly 60 percent, from twenty-four to ten migraines a year. In addition, among the 111 subjects who obtained substantial benefits, 24 stopped having migraines. These results exceed those seen with many migraine drugs.

Other substantial improvements were seen in migraine duration, and degree of nausea and vomiting accompanying migraines. Treatment also reduced the need for other migraine medication. These improvements were statistically significant.

You may wonder which oil was most responsible for these excellent results. Most likely, it was the GLA. There is scant evidence that alpha linolenic acid benefits migraines.

What the Research Tells Us

The research suggesting GLA's effectiveness as migraine therapy is limited but impressive. Unfortunately, the amount of GLA used in the previously mentioned study is not clear, but high dosages of this fatty acid have been known to provide successful results in the treatment of other medical conditions, particularly rheumatoid arthritis.

Dosage

In studies of people with rheumatoid arthritis, GLA has demonstrated the ability to significantly reduce pain and inflammation. In this research, dosages of 1500 to 2400 mg of GLA were used. If you are getting your GLA from such sources as evening primrose oil supplements, it would take a lot of pills to reach this high dosage, as only 10 percent of the oil derived from evening primrose is made of GLA. For example, if you obtain a supplement with 1500 mg of evening primrose oil, you would have to take ten to fourteen pills a day to get 1500 mg of GLA. Because this is a large amount of pills, check with an alternative health care professional for guidance.

GLA works slowly. In the arthritis studies, it took six to twelve months for patients to experience the complete benefits of this therapy. Adverse effects were few and mild, and included abdominal pain, tension headache, nausea, and loose stools. Be aware that GLA may also increase the risk of seizures slightly in people who are prone to this disorder. If this concern applies to you, check with your doctor before taking GLA. If you are taking prescription medication, check with your pharmacist regarding possible unwanted interactions with GLA.

4. MIND AND BODY REMEDIES

Some people prefer to treat medical conditions such as migraines with a mind-body approach rather than by taking substances such as vitamins, herbs, or pharmaceutical medications. Biofeedback and acupuncture have been proven to improve migraine disorder and do not require the ingestion of any substances. These mind-body remedies may be particularly useful to people who are highly sensitive to chemicals and who may react poorly to pills or supplements, even if they are naturally derived.

BIOFEEDBACK

Biofeedback is a behavioral therapy in which subjects learn techniques to attain deep relaxation and control certain physiological functions. It can teach individuals how to influence such processes as skin temperature, heart rate, and even the frequency of brain waves. The ability to manipulate these mechanisms can, in turn, lead to a reduction of physical or mental symptoms such as pain, anxiety, stress, as well as an increase in general health. The use of biofeedback to treat migraines has been studied for four decades.

How It Works

Biofeedback was conceived in the 1950s during research experiments that trained animals to manifest involuntary, or autonomic, bodily responses to external stimuli, similar to how Pavlov trained dogs to salivate at the sound of a bell ringing. If animals could learn to salivate on command, scientists thought, perhaps humans could learn to alter certain autonomic physiological processes, if provided with the proper cues.

Biofeedback utilizes precise instruments to measure activities controlled by the autonomic nervous system, such as muscle tension and skin temperature. A small sensor placed on the scalp or finger conveys data to the biofeedback machine, which displays subtle changes in these activities on a monitor that patients view. At the same time, a biofeedback therapist provides instruction on how to relax the mind and body. By doing so, patients can see how these relaxation techniques may reduce or increase specific physiological processes such as muscle tone or skin temperature. Although the monitor reflects only changes in scalp or finger, alterations also occur in other parts of the body. These changes can reduce symptoms of many conditions including migraines.

Although biofeedback is learned in a therapist's office, it also can be practiced at home. Monitors can be purchased inexpensively. Once learned, individuals can use biofeedback to relieve stress, promote relaxation and sleep, and assist in the treatment of medical conditions such as high blood pressure and migraines. It is a technique that can be helpful for the rest of the user's life.

Scientific Reports of Biofeedback's Effectiveness

While most of the research listed here was conducted recently, biofeedback has been considered a potential migraine remedy ever since scientists stumbled upon its ability to relieve these headaches over forty years ago.

● **1972 (First Report).** At the Menninger Foundation in 1971, a research subject of Dr. Elmer Green was learning biofeedback methods to increase the warmth of her hands.[1] As she gradually increased the blood flow in her hands to warm them, a migraine she was having disappeared. Two other research subjects with migraines soon volunteered for the same training. One obtained complete relief from a migraine, and the other achieved partial relief.

Because of these promising results, Dr. Green and Dr. Joseph Sargent undertook a study that used biofeedback training to treat migraines. As they had in their previous study, the researchers taught their subjects how to increase the temperature of their hands through the use of biofeedback. The technique was formally taught on a weekly basis, and subjects also practiced it at home. After a month, the formal teaching ended, but the subjects continued to use biofeedback at home every other day.

The results of this study were rated by three researchers—an internist and two psychologists. The internist rated twenty-nine of the thirty-two patients (90 percent) as improved. Of the two psychologists, one rated twenty-six of the subjects (80 percent) as improved, while the other concluded the same of twenty-two of the patients (68 percent). These excellent results far exceeded the benefits of medications available then, and continue to exceed the benefits of medications available now.

The doctors commented, "It is important to point out that the patients came to the project because of the inability of other therapeutic modalities to help them. Some of the patients had histories of considerable disability from headaches going back many, many years. If autogenic feedback training [biofeedback] truly has something significant to offer, it is exactly this group of headache sufferers who should benefit the most."

Migraine sufferers who have not improved with migraine drugs or other remedies drugs can be very difficult to treat successfully. The results in this study—improvements of 68 to 90 percent—were not only far beyond expectations, but occurred in a group of subjects that are usually resistant to treatment.

● **2005.** Propranolol is an effective prescription medication used to prevent migraines. In this study, ninety-six longtime migraine sufferers were treated with 80 mg of propranolol every day for six months, while another ninety-six migraineurs were treated with biofeedback daily for the same period of time. Biofeedback subjects were taught muscle relaxation and deep breathing exercises, and their response was measured by relaxation of the frontalis muscle of the forehead and by increases in temperature of the middle finger of their dominant hand.[2]

Both groups experienced a sharp and significant reduction in migraine frequency. After six months of treatment, the biofeedback group saw the occurrence of migraines drop 67 percent on average, while the propranolol group obtained a 65-percent average decrease. The results were virtually identical.

Improvements in migraine duration and severity were also seen in both groups. With propranolol, average migraine duration dropped from fifteen to nine hours, and average severity fell from level four to level two. In the biofeedback group, average migraine duration decreased from fifteen to eight hours, and severity level dropped from four to two.

Although both groups yielded similar findings, a greater percentage of biofeedback subjects rated their outcomes as excellent (an improvement of 76 to 100 percent) or good (an improvement of 51 to 75 percent). Among the patients that used biofeedback, the best results were obtained with relaxation therapy using peripheral temperature monitoring of the finger.

Equally important to this study's conclusions were the outcomes of both groups one year later. At this point, 53 percent of the propranolol subjects reported a resurgence of their migraines. In comparison, only 9 percent of the biofeedback subjects experienced a resurgence of their migraines. This difference was statistically significant. It was also important because it proved the long-term benefits of biofeedback therapy.

Biofeedback also produced fewer side effects than propranolol. Thirteen propranolol subjects (14 percent) experienced adverse reactions, whereas only 4 biofeedback patients (4 percent) noticed side effects.

The researchers concluded, "It is recommended that biofeedback assisted breathing and systematic relaxation should be routinely used for prophylaxis of migraine with or without conventional medicines." They added that biofeedback therapy "had a significantly better long-term prophylactic effect than propranolol in migraine."

● **2010.** Thirty-seven people with long histories of migraines were treated with biofeedback for six months in this prospective study.[3] Each subject had used many different drugs to prevent migraines prior to this research. The patients' ages ranged from nine to seventy-nine. The group included eight people aged fifty-five or older, and eight youngsters between the ages of nine and fifteen. Twenty-nine of the subjects were women.

Subjects used both thermal biofeedback (taking the temperature of the middle finger) and a new method called neurofeedback, which places tiny electrodes on the scalp over various lobes of the brain, starting with the temporal lobe. With this method, the subject can gradually alter brain wave activity, changing highly active rhythms to calmer ones. Because abnormal brain wave activity has been found in migraine sufferers, the researchers sought to discover whether neurofeedback might be effective in the prevention these headaches.

Considerable success was obtained with these biofeedback methods. At baseline, subjects averaged 7.6 migraines per month. After treatment, migraine frequency dropped to 2.9 per month—an improvement of 62 percent. An overall breakdown of the findings reveals that, of the thirty-seven subjects, nine (24 percent) reported an improvement of 50 to 74 percent, eleven (30 percent) noted an improvement of 75 to 95 percent, and four (11 percent) improved 100 percent (no migraines). In other words, 69 percent of subjects felt their migraines reduced by 50 percent or more with biofeedback. These results were excellent and statistically significant. Another seven participants experienced some benefits from therapy, and only six subjects did not improve at all.

The patients were interviewed up to two years after treatment was discontinued. Amazingly, 62 percent continued to enjoy a major or total reduction in migraine frequency. Many subjects also described improvement in other areas. Two-thirds of the group (67 percent) reported a decrease in anxiety or depression, or an increase in focus and concentration, and 55 percent experienced improved sleep.

Additional Evidence

There are many more studies that demonstrate biofeedback's ability to effectively treat migraines. Instead of listing each one, I will cite an extensive review of biofeedback studies that was conducted by Nestoriuc and Martin and published in the medical journal *Pain* in 2007. Based on their in-depth search of major medical databases, including Medline, the Cochrane Library, and others, they examined fifty-five high-quality studies of the use of biofeedback as migraine therapy. Their analysis determined that "behavioral migraine treatments have consistently shown biofeedback to be effective, with average improvement rates around 40 percent and with clinical reductions in migraine activity equaling those of pharmacotherapies."[4] In other words, biofeedback was as helpful as prescription drugs in the treatment of migraine headaches.

These researchers concluded, "Biofeedback significantly and substantially reduces the pain and psychological symptoms of [long-term migraine] patients within the scope of only 11 sessions. Thus, biofeedback can be recommended as an evidence-based behavioral treatment option for the prevention of migraine."

Finally, a 2011 case report from The Peoples' Pharmacy makes a very convincing argument for biofeedback as migraine therapy:

> I was getting migraines several times per week (mostly triggered by stress) for about 8 years—almost every day at one point. After a few months of biofeedback combined with massage therapy I am down to a few per month (generally triggered by PMS). In addition to learning how to control my breathing/tension/stress at biofeedback, I also learned to adjust other parts of my life (i.e. exercise—VERY important!, more protein, consistent sleep pattern).[5]

Compelling testimonials such as this one are excellent additions to the body of evidence that supports the role of biofeedback in migraine treatment.

What the Research Tell Us

Even by rigorous medical standards, the evidence for the effectiveness of biofeedback in the treatment of migraines is strong. Nevertheless, biofeedback does have a few drawbacks. It takes time to do and costs substantially more than most natural supplements and many prescription drugs. On the other hand, biofeedback rarely causes adverse effects. And unlike medications, biofeedback training usually requires only five to ten sessions, in contrast to pills that you may need to take for the rest of your life.

Moreover, biofeedback training can produce other benefits. Its techniques can reduce stress and anxiety, lower blood pressure, and help facilitate sleep. Although the upfront costs of biofeedback are high, it may still be one of the best overall bargains in migraine treatment when its many advantages are considered. If provided by a licensed therapist, bio-feedback may even be covered by your health insurance provider.

ACUPUNCTURE

Acupuncture is an alternative health treatment that uses needles inserted into a patient's skin to bring the body's flow of energy back into balance. For over three thousand years, acupuncture has been a thera-peutic mainstay in traditional Chinese medicine. In many countries today, acupuncture is frequently used to prevent migraines.

How It Works

According to traditional Chinese medicine, energy flows through the body along pathways called merid-ians, and health conditions occur when this energy is disrupted. By stimulating certain acupuncture points along the appropriate meridians, acupuncture is meant to correct the flow of energy along these pathways and heal illness. Although these points and meridians have never been shown to exist scientifically, current theory suggests that acupuncture needles may trigger nerves in a manner that reduces pain and other signs of medical illness.

Scientific Reports of Acupuncture's Effectiveness

Anecdotal stories about the benefits of acupuncture have existed for thousands of years. This first scientific report, however, is the earliest evidence available in US medical literature. It is likely, though, that Chinese medical literature contains many earlier articles attesting to acupuncture's effectiveness in the prevention of migraines.

● **1992 (First Report).** Over a ten-year span, Dr. Z. Pingping treated forty-seven patients who experienced chronic migraines.[6] Thirty-two of the subjects were women. The patients' ages ranged from seventeen to sixty-two, and their migraine attacks lasted between three days and two weeks. The doctor reported, "Among the 47 patients, 32 were cured with 1 session of acupuncture treatment, 11 after 2 sessions, and 3 patients after 3 sessions." (One patient quit treatment after one session without follow-up.)

In one case, a twenty-seven-year-old woman came to the doctor with a migraine that had been affecting her for two weeks. Previous attempts to cure it with medications and Chinese herbs had failed. The woman received two acupuncture treatments over a span of two days, and subsequently had no further migraines during the six months of follow-up.

In another case, a thirty-two-year-old man was suffering severe migraines on the left side of his head during sleep but not during the day. An acupuncture treatment given one hour prior to sleep prevented him from having a migraine that night and each subsequent night.

● **1994.** In a randomized, placebo-controlled study, acupuncture was compared with the beta-blocker drug metoprolol and a placebo known as fake acupuncture, which uses random points on the body (also called sham acupuncture).[7] Fake acupuncture was used to insure that the power of suggestion was not the cause of improvement. Acupuncture and metoprolol proved significantly superior remedies to the placebo, and were equally effective in reducing migraine frequency and duration. Metoprolol was modestly more effective than acupuncture in lowering migraine severity, whereas acupuncture caused fewer side effects than the medication.

● **2006.** For those who demand big drug company-style studies, here is a prospective, randomized, multicenter, double-blind, parallel-group, controlled clinical trial. It involved 960 subjects who were having two to six migraines per month.[8] Subjects received ten sessions of either traditional acupuncture or sham acupuncture. A third group received medication to prevent migraines.

After twenty-six weeks, all groups obtained a significant reduction in migraine frequency compared to baseline. The groups that received acupuncture or standard medication obtained greater benefits than the sham acupuncture patients. Interestingly, 47 percent of subjects in the actual acupuncture group noted a drop in migraine frequency of 50 percent or better. Furthermore, 40 percent of the medication group saw the same degree of migraine reduction, while 39 percent of sham acupuncture subjects obtained similar results. Actual acupuncture proved superior to both metoprolol and sham acupuncture.

● **2006.** In another randomized, controlled, multi-center trial that extended over twenty-four weeks, acupuncture was compared again with the beta-blocker medication metoprolol in the prevention of chronic migraines.[9] On average, the acupuncture patients obtained a 42 percent reduction in migraine occurrence, while the metoprolol group's migraine frequency dropped 38 percent. Impressively, 61 percent of acupuncture subjects attained a 50-percent or greater decrease in migraine attacks, while 49 percent of metoprolol patients saw the same level of improvement.

Not only was acupuncture superior to metoprolol in its ability to prevent migraines, but it also caused fewer side effects. Only two of the fifty-nine acupuncture patients (4 percent) withdrew from treatment, whereas eighteen of the fifty-five metoprolol patients (33 percent) left the study. Clearly, side effects were far fewer and milder for the subjects receiving acupuncture than those taking the prescription drug.

The following table outlines the results of this study.

Treatment	Average Improvement	50 % or Greater Improvement	Quit Treatment Due to Side Effects
Acupuncture	42 %	61 %	4 %
Metoprolol	38 %	49 %	33 %

● **2009.** A major review by the highly respected Cochrane Collaboration in England thoroughly assessed the effectiveness of acupuncture in migraine prevention.[10] The Cochrane review encompassed twenty-two acupuncture studies, which had a total number of 4419 participants. It included two large trials—one that included 1715 participants and the other that included 401.

In six studies that compared acupuncture with standard migraine therapy (prescription or over-the-counter drugs) and no treatment, acupuncture showed superior effectiveness and was associated with fewer headaches than the other methods. In four other studies that contrasted acupuncture therapy with medications used to prevent migraines, acupuncture produced equal or better results and had fewer side effects.

The authors of the review concluded, "Available studies suggest that acupuncture is at least as effective as, or possibly more effective than, prophylactic drug treatment, and has fewer adverse effects. Acupuncture should be considered a treatment option for patients willing to undergo this treatment."

What the Research Tells Us

There are many additional studies of acupuncture as a migraine treatment. Most were published recently, and most demonstrated significant benefits of this method. Only a few did not. When researched along-side common migraine drugs, acupuncture has proven to be equally or slightly more effective than pharmaceuticals in the prevention of migraines, and far less likely to cause side effects.

5. PREVENTING MIGRAINES IN CHILDREN AND ADOLESCENTS

Migraines affect 3 to 10 percent of children, with the incidence increasing with age to nearly 20 percent in older adolescents. Migraines occur in an equal number of girls and boys during childhood, but afflict twice as many girls as boys by late adolescence. Puberty brings an end to these headaches in some children, while adolescence sometimes marks the first appearance of this disorder in others. Unfortunately, many teenagers with migraines continue to have them as adults.

While an adult will generally experience migraine pain on only one side of the head, a child's migraine is often bilateral or located in the middle of the forehead. The attacks are frequently accompanied by sensitivity to noise or light and can last one to seventy-two hours.

Children may also experience conditions thought to be equivalent to migraines. These include abdominal migraines (in which the pain is located in the belly and can cause nausea and vomiting), recurrent attacks of vertigo, and severe neck spasms. These conditions can be difficult to diagnose because there are no

abnormal findings during an attack except for pain. A
diagnosis of a migraine equivalent should be considered for a youngster who has a severely painful,
episodic disorder that displays normal medical test
results during an attack, yet causes no pain and shows
no abnormal medical findings between episodes. Dr.
Larry Romane, an emergency room specialist, says
that the most common causes of episodic abdominal
pain in a child are chronic constipation or abdominal
migraine. (Interestingly, magnesium can treat both.)

It is vitally important to identify children with
migraines, not only to provide them with pain relief,
but also because such children often have sleep disorders and display poor school performance. Thus, a
child with undiagnosed and untreated migraines may
experience lifelong under-achievement and low self-
esteem. Once a diagnosis of migraines is made, however, many parents have mixed feelings about
traditional treatment with pharmaceuticals. While
they want their child to feel better, they are also con-
cerned about the side effects of migraine drugs and
the long-term impact these side effects might have on
a growing young person. Thankfully, a handful of the
natural remedies mentioned in this book have demonstrated the ability to prevent migraines in children
and adolescents. Listed in descending order of effectiveness, the following treatments may provide help
to numerous young migraine sufferers.

5-HYDROXYTRYPTOPHAN (5-HTP)

The first study of 5-HTP's effectiveness in the prevention of migraine headaches in adults came in 1973 and

showed excellent results. A little over a decade later, this bioidentical remedy was put to the test in children.

● **1984.** A double-blind, cross-over study of thirty children with migraine headaches compared 5-HTP therapy with a placebo. The average age of the children was ten. Over twelve weeks, fifteen of the subjects received 100 mg of 5-HTP per day, while the remaining fifteen were given a placebo. The groups then switched, or "crossed over," treatments, and therapy continued for an additional twelve weeks.

When a group received 5-HTP, its members experienced reductions in the migraine index, which is a combined measurement of migraine frequency, severity, and duration. Compared with placebo, the improvements with 5-HTP therapy were substantial and scientifically significant.[1]

● **1987.** In a double-blind, placebo-controlled study, forty-eight elementary school students with a history of migraines and sleep disorders received 5-HTP in a dosage of 4.5 mg/kg (milligrams per kilogram), or approximately 2 mg/lb (milligrams per pound), or a placebo every day for eight weeks. Treatment was then crossed over for another eight weeks.

Therapy with 5-HTP reduced the migraine index by 70 percent, yet the placebo produced only an 11.5-percent decrease. This result was scientifically significant. Sleep also improved in the 5-HTP group. Finally, no side effects were reported with the use of 5-HTP.[2]

BUTTERBUR

Because previous studies had demonstrated the effectiveness of butterbur extract in adult migraine prevention, a study was undertaken in 2005 to determine whether this natural remedy might also help children with migraine headaches.[3]

● **2005.** This research included 108 subjects between the ages of eight and twelve. Children nine years old and under received 50 to 75 mg of butterbur extract each day for four months, while those ten years old and above received 100 to 150 mg daily. On average, the group had been experiencing migraines for two and a half years.

The subjects demonstrated significant improvement as a result of butterbur therapy, with 77 percent of them obtaining a reduction in migraine frequency of 50 percent or greater. On average, migraine attacks decreased 63 percent.

Substantial benefits were reported by 79 percent of subjects or their parents. Another 10 percent described modest improvements. Migraine duration fell from an average of ten hours prior to treatment to seven hours with butterbur therapy. Overall, 63 percent of the children experienced a reduction in migraine duration. In a few subjects, however, migraine duration increased.

Nearly 90 percent of the doctors noted positive results in the children who received butterbur treatment. Only seven of the study's subjects reported adverse effects. None were serious or necessitated withdrawal from the research. The most common side effect was burping, which occurred in four of the children.

The researchers concluded, "Butterbur root extract shows potential as an effective and well-tolerated migraine prophylaxis also for children and teenagers."

COENZYME Q$_{10}$

In a clinic for migraine sufferers who had not improved with standard medical treatment, blood levels of CoQ_{10} were tested in children and adolescents. Interestingly, more than half of the youngsters were found to have low levels of CoQ_{10}.[4] In light of this finding, a study was conducted to determine the effectiveness of CoQ_{10} supplementation in the prevention of migraine attacks in young people.

● **2005.** This research included 252 subjects of an average age of thirteen, all of whom had low CoQ_{10} levels. Two-thirds of the patients were female. The group's headache frequency was high, averaging nineteen days per month.

The subjects received CoQ_{10} in dosages of 1 to 3 mg/kg every day, depending on age. On average, blood levels of CoQ_{10} improved from a pre-study level of 0.46 mcg/mL (micrograms per milliliter) to a normal level of 1.2 mcg/mL after CoQ_{10} treatment—a nearly threefold increase.

Supplementation with CoQ_{10} caused the average frequency of migraines to drop from nineteen days to twelve and a half days per month—a 34-percent reduction. Moreover, 46 percent of the subjects obtained a 50-percent or greater decrease in migraine occurrence, matching the standard medical definition of treatment success for migraines.

The researchers concluded, "Given the high frequency of CoQ_{10} deficiency and relatively low potential side effects, all [migraine] patients may benefit from CoQ_{10} supplementation."

MELATONIN

Only a few years after melatonin was first reported as an effective migraine treatment in adults, fourteen children were selected consecutively at a headache center to test whether melatonin might reduce these headaches in younger people.[5] Personally, I like the model of choosing patients consecutively, as it avoids the selection biases that can often be seen in more elaborate research. The population treated in this study was likely typical of those seen in many doctors' offices.

● **2008.** This study was open-label. The children, parents, and doctors knew the treatment was 3 mg of melatonin at bedtime. There was no placebo group. Instead, the frequency, severity, and duration of migraines with melatonin were compared with baseline measurements taken a month before melatonin therapy began.

Of the thirteen children who completed the study, ten (77 percent) obtained a reduction in migraine frequency of greater than 50 percent. This result was statistically significant and medically impressive. Migraine duration and intensity also dropped 25 to 30 percent on average. Equally important to note is the fact that melatonin did not cause a worsening of migraines in any subject.

The doctors concluded, "In our small series of children with primary headache [migraine or tension], melatonin effectively reduced the number, intensity and duration of headache attacks per month. Our results in children confirm published reports ascribing the benefit of melatonin prophylaxis in adult patients."

Only one side effect occurred, which was sedation; and that only happened to one subject. Although this child was sedated by 3 mg of melatonin, a lower dosage could be tried in a real-life situation. Melatonin can be purchased in several dosages, including 0.5, 1, 2, 3, as well as 5 mg.

Whether it is used by adults or children, melatonin can cause sedation. Indeed, it is the chemical made by the body to induce sleep, so it should be taken just before bedtime.

RIBOFLAVIN

Although riboflavin first displayed its ability to prevent migraine headaches in adults in 1946, this vitamin only recently underwent testing to see if it would be an effective therapy for young migraineurs.

● **2009.** This study took place at a specialty clinic for young migraine sufferers who had not responded to standard drug treatment.[6] The subjects had already proven tough to treat and resistant to placebo effects. It was an excellent population in which to test the effectiveness of a natural remedy rigorously.

Twenty-one girls and sixteen boys participated in this outpatient research. They ranged in age from nine to eighteen and averaged two severe migraines a month. The subjects took either 200 or 400 mg of riboflavin each day with breakfast for up to six months.

After three months of riboflavin therapy, 60 percent of subjects obtained a decrease in migraine frequency of 50 percent or more. After six months, 68 percent of subjects claimed the same results—in other words, two-thirds of the group. An additional 18 percent of participants saw their migraine occurrence reduced by 25 to 50 percent. Of children under twelve years of age, 92 percent achieved this degree of improvement.

The average number of days with migraines also dropped after three months of riboflavin therapy—from twenty per month before treatment to thirteen per month. After six months of riboflavin treatment, this number fell to eight migraine days per month, amounting to a total decrease of 65 percent. Both of these findings were highly significant.

The study also measured changes in migraine intensity, which fell 20 percent after three months of riboflavin treatment. After six months, this measurement rose to 30 percent. These results were also statistically significant.

All of these results far exceed those usually seen with prescription drugs. Side effects were seen in only two subjects (5 percent). One participant developed nausea and vomiting due to the unpleasant taste of the riboflavin compound. Another reported increased appetite, although no weight gain was seen.

The doctors summarized their results by stating, "In conclusion, riboflavin seems to be a well-tolerated, effective, and low-cost prophylactic treatment in children and adolescents suffering from migraine." They added, "Riboflavin may be effective for any type of migraine, with any age of onset, in children and adolescents."

GINKGO BILOBA

Ginkgo biloba remains one of the most popular supplements in the country because of its ability to boost memory. The following study is the first to measure ginkgo's effectiveness as a remedy for migraines in both adults and children.

● **2010.** In this study, twenty-four subjects between the ages of eight and eighteen received a combination remedy that contained 80 mg of ginkgo, 20 mg of coenzyme Q_{10}, 1.6 mg of riboflavin, and 300 mg of magnesium twice a day for three months. The subjects had dealt with migraines for more than three years on average, experiencing migraines approximately nine days a month and using prescription migraine medication six times a month.

Preliminary results indicated that the number of migraine days dropped from 7.4 per month at baseline to 2.2 with this therapy—an improvement of 70 percent. Average medication use decreased from 5.9 to 1.5 times per month—a mean reduction of 75 percent.[7,8]

The authors commented, "These preliminary data show that ginkgolide B seems to be effective as preventive treatment in reducing migraine attack frequency and in attenuating the use of symptomatic medication in our small series of children with primary [migraine] headache."

The findings of this study are encouraging, but whether the useful substance was ginkgo or one of the other supplements involved is not known. The dosages of coenzyme Q_{10} and riboflavin were small, but magnesium can have a preventative effect on migraines at 600 mg per day. Still, ginkgo has displayed an ability to inhibit adult migraines on its own and is worth consideration.

WHAT THE RESEARCH TELLS US

As the previously listed studies demonstrate, there are many natural therapies that can help prevent migraines in children and adolescents. When treating children, I always advise caution in the selection of treatments and recommend that families work with their doctors. I suggest starting all remedies at a low dosage, and advise beginning with the bioidentical remedies (5-HTP, coenzyme Q_{10}, melatonin, riboflavin) because of their greater safety profiles. Be especially careful with herbs, which, like prescription drugs, are foreign to human systems and may therefore provoke side effects.

6. Natural Remedies for Acute Migraines

Whether they develop suddenly or gradually, at their peak, migraines cause severe pain and force sufferers to retreat to quiet, darkened rooms due to their intense sensitivity to sound and light. Migraine pain is remarkably powerful and disables millions of sufferers. It is often more than aspirin, nonsteroidal anti-inflammatory drugs (NSAIDs), or acetaminophen can handle. Sleep brings relief to some migraine victims, but not to others.

Only a few therapies are capable of halting an acute migraine. In mainstream medicine, drugs from the triptan family, such as sumatriptan (Imitrex), rizatriptan (Maxalt), and zolmitriptan (Zomig), are frequently prescribed for acute migraine attacks because of their ability to quickly shrink swollen blood vessels in the brain. These drugs are taken orally or as a nasal spray. Minor side effects can occur, including abnormal sensations (4 percent), chest tightness (2 percent), dizziness (6 percent), dry flushing (5 percent), hot and cold sensations (5 percent), nausea (7 percent), and weakness (7 percent). More serious side effects occur infrequently.

In emergency rooms, sumatriptan (Imitrex) is often injected subcutaneously. It works fast, but as its manufacturer warns, it can cause heart attacks and death. Other possible side effects include injection site reaction (59 percent), atypical sensations (42 percent), tingling (14 percent), dizziness (12 percent), warm or hot sensation (11 percent), burning sensation (7 percent), feeling of pressure (7 percent), flushing (7 percent), feeling numbness (5 percent), weakness (5 percent), and sweating (2 percent).

With these potential side effects, why would anyone want to take a triptan drug before trying a natural remedy? Why would any doctor, especially an emergency room doctor, prescribe a triptan before attempting a natural therapy? Consider this: Only half of people who receive a triptan drug for an acute migraine become pain-free. Many of the natural remedies described below work just as well as pharmaceuticals and have fewer risks. In fact, there are six natural therapies—magnesium, niacin, riboflavin, vitamin D, ginger, and acupuncture—that have been shown to halt acute migraines.

MAGNESIUM

Magnesium's ability to halt acute migraines was first reported in an article published almost a century ago. Since then, this bioidentical remedy has proven to be as effective as migraine drugs and should be considered a first-line therapy when these headaches strike.

● **1933.** As noted in "Magnesium" on page 35, an article in the highly respected medical journal *Lancet* described the treatment of a thirty-two-year-old woman who had suffered for years from severe nocturnal migraines accompanied by vomiting and palpitations. They wrote, "A dozen injections of magnesium sulphate cut short the attacks and she now has been free from them for a year."[1] Although the authors did not explain whether the injections were intravenous or intramuscular, nor did they mention the dosage of magnesium used, her improvement was remarkable. The woman's long-term recovery was likely due to a sustained elevation of magnesium in her tissues.

● **1995.** Nationally respected magnesium researchers Alexander Mauskop and Burt and Bella Altura published a study in which they treated forty consecutive acute migraine sufferers with 1,000 mg of magnesium sulfate intravenously.[2] I like this type of study because it reflects exactly what doctors encounter in offices and emergency rooms.

In thirty-five of the subjects (88 percent), pain reduction of 50 percent or more occurred within fifteen minutes of infusion. In twenty-one patients (53 percent), pain relief persisted for twenty-four hours or longer, a result that many prescription medications cannot match.

When the patients began the study, blood was drawn and magnesium levels were measured by an advanced test not currently available in medical laboratories. Pain relief lasted at least twenty-four hours in 86 percent of subjects with low magnesium levels, yet in only 16 percent of those with normal magnesium levels. These findings suggest that magnesium can be highly effective in the treatment of migraines in people with magnesium deficiencies, but much less so in those with normal magnesium levels.

You would think a simple blood test would differentiate people with magnesium deficiency from those with adequate magnesium. Standard magnesium blood tests, however, are not highly accurate, and many people with normal lab test results are actually deficient in this mineral. The most reliable test is simply to take magnesium and see if it works.

● **2001.** In this randomized, placebo-controlled study published in 2001, fifteen patients received 1,000 mg of magnesium sulfate intravenously over a fifteen-minute period.[3] The next fifteen patients received a standard intravenous salt solution as a placebo. If pain persisted after thirty minutes in the placebo group, those patients were then given intravenous magnesium.

Of the fifteen patients who received magnesium initially, thirteen (87 percent) experienced complete elimination of pain, while two had partial relief. Other symptoms such as nausea and light sensitivity disappeared in all fifteen people. In comparison, only one subject in the placebo group experienced any decrease in pain. After thirty minutes, all placebo subjects were given intravenous magnesium. All improved. In fact, migraine attacks ceased in fourteen (93 percent) of them. The results of this study are powerful as well as scientifically significant.

The doctors concluded, "Our results show that 1,000 mg of intravenous magnesium sulfate is an efficient, safe, and well tolerated drug in the treatment of migraine attacks."

● **2002.** Migraine patients with and without aura symptoms (light sensitivity, sound sensitivity, irritability, and nausea) were compared in a double-blind, placebo-controlled study that used 1,000 mg of intravenous magnesium sulfate to treat acute migraines.

Migraineurs without auras obtained only slight benefits from magnesium therapy when compared with
placebo. Yet, in the patients with aura symptoms,
intravenous magnesium produced significant improvements in comparison to placebo.[4]

● **Note.** The oral dosage of magnesium needed to halt
an impending migraine has not been established. The
Recommended Daily Intake of magnesium is 400 mg,
but larger amounts have been used in several studies.
(See "Magnesium" on page 35.) To prevent acute
migraines, many of the recently mentioned reports
employed 1,000 mg of magnesium intravenously. This
type of treatment would have to be administered in a
doctor's office or an emergency room. Intravenous
magnesium therapy is well known in some hospital
settings, such as cardiac and maternity intensive care
units.

NIACIN

Like magnesium, niacin is a bioidentical migraine
remedy that has a long history of scientific evidence to
support it. Reports of its ability to halt acute migraines
go back decades. Under the proper medical supervi-
sion, niacin can be an impressive treatment when a
migraine threatens to take hold.

● **1944.** In a study reported in the *Annals of Internal
Medicine,* Dr. Miles Atkinson treated twenty-one
patients who had been suffering from migraines for
many years. Using various combinations of intravenous, intramuscular, and oral niacin, seventeen
patients (81 percent) reported substantial improve-

ments. Some subjects even noted immediate relief with an injection of niacin.[5]

● **1949.** In the May volume of *The American Practitioner,* Dr. R.F. Grenfell reported the use of intravenous niacin in dosages of 100 to 300 mg to treat acute migraines. The niacin was administered to fifteen people during thirty-one severe migraine attacks. All of the subjects had already failed to benefit from migraine drugs. Niacin was beneficial in twenty-seven cases (87 percent).[6]

The majority of this study's subjects received a dosage of 100 mg, and most others were given 200 mg. Only two patients required 300 mg. Dr. Grenfell used enough niacin to produce flushing sensations in all subjects. He described these reactions as "uncomfortable sensations of tingling and burning of the skin, [although] no patient objected strenuously to the treatment." No subject reported any worsening of their migraines.

● **1991.** J.A. Hall reported his successful use of oral niacin to abort acute migraine attacks. He noted that improvement began at the same time that intense flushing from the niacin occurred.[7,8]

● **2001.** In the journal *Medical Hypotheses,* psychologist Dr. A. Gedye suggested an unusual combination of natural substances to halt acute migraines: tryptophan, calcium, caffeine, aspirin, and niacin.[9] Dr. Gedye reasoned that aspirin (or naproxen) would reduce inflammation; caffeine and calcium would reduce the vasodilation that occurs in the blood vessels of the brain during migraines; tryptophan would restore reduced blood levels of serotonin, which are reduced during migraines; and niacin would prevent tryptophan from being shunted to other systems, thereby maintaining the increased serotonin levels from the tryptophan.

Dr. Gedye tested this combination in twelve subjects, eight of whom were women, who had histories of long-term, chronic migraines. The therapy contained 500 mg of tryptophan, 100 mg of regular niacin, 500 mg of calcium carbonate, 64 mg of caffeine (equal to less than 1 cup of coffee), and 650 mg of aspirin (one regular aspirin pill).

The subjects were not told of the ingredients and agreed to take the therapy at the beginning of their next ten migraines. They were also told to avoid foods or supplements with high levels of potassium or magnesium, which might increase vasodilation. They were allowed to take a second dose if the migraine returned after four hours. If the second dose was not helpful, they were instructed to take a non-sedating antihistamine (such as Claritin).

Nine of the twelve (75 percent) subjects responded well to this approach, obtaining complete or nearly complete cessation of acute migraines. Because of their good results, they continued to use the treatment successfully for two more years. No side effects were reported.

The substances used by Dr. Gedye can be obtained in their specified dosages without a prescription. Regular niacin at a dosage of 100 mg may cause mild flushing in some people.

● **2002.** In an article in the *Journal of Orthomolecular Medicine*, Dr. Jonathan Prousky and Dr. Erika Sykes described the responses of two people who took oral niacin for acute migraine relief.[10] In the first case, a thirty-two-year-old man had been suffering from migraines once a week for twelve years. He described his migraines as a constant stabbing pain that lasted all day. The doctor gave him 500 mg of oral niacin, which caused a full-body flush in thirty to forty-five minutes, but also resulted in the man reporting partial relief from the migraine attack. After another thirty minutes, the migraine disappeared. He took niacin on three similar occasions, and each time the niacin aborted his acute migraine.

In the second case, a twenty-seven-year-old man received 500 mg of niacin for an acute migraine. He felt the niacin flush after thirty minutes, and shortly thereafter also experienced complete relief from his headache.

These cases confirmed the 1991 report by Hall, which stated that niacin was effective for halting acute migraine attacks. They also supported the idea that relief coincides with the development of a niacin flush.

● **Note.** Side effects sometimes occur with niacin that people find unpleasant, including intense flushing and itching of the skin. In fact, about 15 percent of one study's subjects found the niacin flush more bothersome than their migraines. Yet the other patients found niacin to be worth taking because of how well it halted their headaches. See "Niacin" on page 53 for information on the various types of prescription, over-the-counter, and natural forms of this substance, and how to use them. Taking niacin can be tricky, and because side effects often occur, I recommend working with a health care practitioner before treating your migraines with this vitamin.

RIBOFLAVIN

Because the body absorbs this vitamin so quickly, riboflavin supplementation can be an effective way to halt acute migraines. As the following report suggests, this natural remedy may be taken daily, with smaller dosages being used whenever you sense an impending migraine.

● **1946.** Published in the *Canadian Medical Journal* a little over a decade after riboflavin was first synthesized, Dr. Clifford Smith described his success in treating long-suffering migraine patients with low doses of riboflavin.[11] One woman who invariably experienced migraines when traveling by train was able to halt a migraine by taking just 5 mg each hour during her journey. In others, hourly doses of riboflavin for five or six hours often stopped acute migraines.

In many of Dr. Smith's patients, riboflavin use yielded maximum benefits only after three to six months of daily use. (See "Riboflavin" on page 21.) Best results may be achieved by using 400 mg of riboflavin daily, with smaller doses such as 25 mg taken hourly to halt an acute migraine.

VITAMIN D

Although vitamin D is produced naturally in the skin after exposure to sunlight, many people are deficient in this substance and may benefit from vitamin D supplementation. While this compound is mainly known for its important role in bone health, it has also shown effectiveness in the treatment of migraines. If you have not already had your vitamin D level tested, it is a good idea to do so at your next annual physical exam.

● **1994.** Dr. Thys-Jacobs reported two cases in which a combination of vitamin D and calcium were effective in reducing the frequency of migraines.[12] One of these cases involved a forty-year-old woman with a thirty-year history of migraines and a ten-year history of premenstrual syndrome. The woman averaged four migraines per month, which each lasted one to three days. The headaches were incapacitating and kept her from her work and night classes. Her vitamin D_3 level was low, and treatment with 1,200 IU of vitamin D_3 and 1,200 mg of calcium per day "resulted in a significant reduction of her migraine headaches as well as PMS symptoms."

Equally important to note is the fact that the woman was able to abort acute migraine attacks by taking her daily vitamin D_3 and immediately chewing and swallowing 1,200 to 1,600 mg of calcium when one was about to strike.

GINGER

Ginger is one of the most common herbal remedies available today. It is widely used and studied for its ability to reduce the nausea and vomiting that can accompany pregnancy and chemotherapy, but is also beginning to be known as a potential treatment for both chronic and acute migraines.

● **2005.** A study underwritten by the manufacturer of GelStat and published in *Medical Science Monitor* involved twenty-nine people who had been experiencing two to eight migraines per month for one year or more. GelStat is a homeopathic remedy for both acute and chronic migraines.[13] It contains small amounts of the herbs ginger and feverfew. Ginger is likely the active ingredient in the case of acute migraine treatment, as other evidence has shown (See "Ginger" on page 83.)

The subjects were instructed to begin taking GelStat as soon as migraine symptoms developed and before they became severe. All twenty-nine subjects experienced migraines during the research, and fourteen of them (48 percent) were pain-free within two hours of taking Gel-Stat. An additional ten subjects (34 percent) reported only a mild migraine after GelStat treatment, which was an improvement over their usual severe migraines.

Overall, seventeen of the twenty-nine patients (59 percent) were satisfied with GelStat therapy. Twelve participants (41 percent) preferred GelStat to their usual migraine medication or felt it was as effective as the pharmaceutical. The authors concluded, "GelStat Migraine is effective as a first line abortive treatment for migraine when initiated early during the mild headache phase."

ACUPUNCTURE

For migraine patients who do not wish to take drugs or supplements to halt acute migraines, acupuncture may be a welcome alternative. This therapy has proven to be as effective as the pharmaceuticals commonly used to stop acute migraines, as the following studies suggest.

● **2003.** Acupuncture therapy was compared with 6 mg of injectable sumatriptan (Imitrex), a potent drug used to halt acute migraines.[14] Both approaches were also compared with an injection of a placebo. Of the sixty subjects, acupuncture prevented a full migraine in twenty-one (35 percent), while sumatriptan prevented a full migraine in twenty-one of fifty-eight patients (36 percent). Placebo stopped a full migraine in only eleven of sixty-one people (18 percent). The results of both acupuncture therapy and sumatriptan treatment were significantly superior to placebo.

An additional injection of sumatriptan provided substantial relief to 80 percent of the subjects who developed a full migraine despite treatment, whereas only 13 percent obtained substantial relief with additional acupuncture. On the other hand, sumatriptan caused side effects in 40 percent of its subjects, while only 24 percent of the acupuncture group experienced adverse reactions. Although serious side effects did not occur in sumatriptan users in this study, injectable sumatriptan is known to cause severe, sometimes life-threatening reactions in a small percentage of people.

Overall, the study demonstrated that acupuncture was as effective as the powerful migraine drug sumatriptan in the prevention of a full migraine, but not as effective as the drug when a second administration was required.

● **2009.** In an effort to halt acute migraine attacks, 175 subjects received true acuptuncture or a placebo of sham acupuncture.[15] The subjects averaged approximately forty years of age, and 60 percent of them were female. They had been experiencing migraines for 3.5 years on average, with migraine histories ranging from 1.5 to 10 years.

At two and four hours after treatment, true acupuncture proved significantly superior to the placebo at reducing migraine pain. In fact, 41 percent of patients who underwent true acupuncture gained complete relief from discomfort. Overall, 30 percent of those who received true acupuncture noted a 75-precent or greater improvement in symptoms.

WHAT THE RESEARCH TELLS US

According to the available evidence, magnesium, niacin, and acupuncture are the most effective and reliable natural remedies for acute migraines. Although the report of riboflavin as a potential acute migraine treatment is limited, the proof of its effectiveness in migraine prevention suggests that it might also stop acute attacks. And while more research on vitamin D and ginger would be useful, they may be used to treat acute migraines regardless, due to their high margins of safety.

If you have found that other natural therapies such as coenzyme Q_{10}, melatonin, or biofeedback greatly reduce the frequency, intensity, or duration of your migraines, you might also try using them to stop an acute migraine. That fact that no study has been published to date on their ability to halt acute attacks does not mean that these remedies will not work for you.

CONCLUSION

Topiramate (Topamax) is a best-selling migraine drug and a favorite of thousands of doctors. Several years ago, a highly respected team of doctors conducted a large placebo-controlled, double-blind, randomized study of 469 subjects to test topiramate's effectiveness in migraine prevention.[1] Migraine frequency was reduced by 39 percent in those who received 100 mg of topiramate, and by 38 percent in those who received 200 mg of the drug. Most of natural remedies in this book, however, top those numbers. For example, in a 1985 study of feverfew, migraine occurrence dropped 80 percent.[2]

Of the topiramate users in this study, 53 percent obtained a 50-percent or greater reduction in monthly migraine frequency. These are good results, but they are matched or exceeded by most of the natural remedies presented in this book. For example, in a study of melatonin's use in the prevention of migraines, 80 percent of subjects achieved a 50-percent or greater decrease in migraine frequency.[3] Furthermore, in a study of butterbur's effect on children's migraines, 77 percent of the children obtained a 50-percent or greater reduction in migraine occurrence.[4]

Moreover, while natural remedies generally provoke very few adverse reactions, topiramate can cause plenty of them, including paresthesias (nerve disturbances), nausea, fatigue, abnormal taste in the mouth, sedation, impaired concentration, impaired memory, and speech and language problems. In this study, the 126 subjects that took 100 mg of topiramate each day reported 169 side effects. That's an average of 1.3 side effects per person. Not surprisingly, nineteen participants (13 percent) quit the study.

The statistics were even worse for the subjects in the group that took 200 mg of topiramate, 113 of which reported 184 side effects. That's an average of 1.6 per person. Furthermore, twenty-six patients (23 percent) withdrew from the study. These are serious numbers, but not surprising ones. In studies of migraine drugs, 30 to 40 percent of participants commonly experience side effects. The rate of people who quit treatment due to adverse reactions to these drugs often approaches 20 percent. By comparison, the natural remedies described in this book cause few side effects, and very few people discontinue treatment when using them.

Considering the fact that topiramate and other drugs like it are likely to result in adverse reactions, and that their benefits are no better than the natural remedies highlighted in this book, are pharmaceuticals really the first therapy you want to try for migraine relief? Is there any question that you should initially consider remedies that are natural, effective, inexpensive, and safer?

THE BEST NATURAL REMEDIES

Based on the studies presented in this book, the following therapies are the best natural remedies for migraine headaches (listed alphabetically).

- Acupuncture

- Biofeedback

- Butterbur

- Coenzyme Q_{10}

- Feverfew

- 5-Hydroxytryptophan

- Magnesium

- Melatonin

- Riboflavin

- White Willow and Feverfew

According to some experts, the natural remedy with the strongest evidence of effectiveness in migraine prevention is butterbur, followed by feverfew, magnesium, riboflavin, coenzyme Q_{10}, and melatonin. On the other hand, feverfew combined with white willow provided the strongest evidence I have seen in a single study of migraine prevention. The study was small, and there are no other studies to corroborate its findings, but feverfew has been established as a migraine remedy on its own, and the proven biochemical activity of white willow gives this herb a strong theoretical basis as a migraine treatment.

Although the other remedies in this book did not make the "best of" list, they are certainly worth trying if the top choices fail. Similarly, although the scientific data was not strong enough to include yoga, meditation, hypnosis, or cognitive behavioral therapy in this book, you might also consider these therapies. As with biofeedback or acupuncture, these other mind-body methods can be tried along with other natural remedies or prescription drugs.

All of the bioidentical remedies outlined in this book can be used alongside prescription or over-the-counter medication. While herbal therapies may be safe for people who also take pharmaceuticals, it is best to check with a doctor or pharmacist about possible herb-drug interactions. Finally, when it comes to stopping acute migraines, the best natural remedies are magnesium, niacin, and riboflavin.

NATURAL REMEDIES IN COMBINATION

Many of the remedies in this book can be taken in combination, particularly the bioidentical ones. Several manufacturers, in fact, make migraine treatments that combine natural substances such as feverfew, magnesium, and riboflavin; or magnesium, riboflavin, butterbur, and coenzyme Q_{10}. Such products make keeping track of individual dosages easier, but you will pay a higher cost for the convenience. In addition, in many of these patented, brand-name combinations of natural remedies, the dosages of the ingredients are too low to be effective.

While a supplement may contain proven remedies such as butterbur, magnesium, and feverfew, it may also include numerous other herbs, many of which may provide questionable benefits. Plus, the more substances you take, the greater the likelihood of an adverse interaction. If you decide to try a combination supplement, start with the lowest recommended dosage, increasing it gradually, if necessary. My recommendation is to combine different remedies individually until you achieve good results. You can do this with many of the natural therapies in this book. For example, you can take the recommended amounts of riboflavin, magnesium, and coenzyme Q_{10} together. Because they are bioidentical, these substances can be mixed with little risk. If necessary, you could add feverfew or butterbur. If simple methods do not work for you, I suggest you consult a knowledgeable integrative or alternative doctor or naturopath for guidance.

RESULTS MAY TAKE TIME

The benefits of many natural remedies only appear after extended use. A natural therapy may produce limited results if taken for only one month, but three to six months of use may deliver an excellent outcome. Give these remedies time to work

If you decide to discontinue an effective remedy, do so gradually. Abrupt discontinuation of any migraine-preventing substance, whether it is a natural remedy or a medication, can trigger rebound migraines. Finally, if you are pregnant, breastfeeding, or trying to become pregnant, ask your doctor before starting any therapy, whether natural or prescription.

YOUR RIGHT OF INFORMED CONSENT

Does your doctor have a responsibility to inform you of natural migraine remedies? Yes! The Code of Medical Ethics states that you need to be informed about all reasonable possibilities in order for you to make reasonable decisions regarding your treatment. This is called *informed consent.*

The American Medical Association Council on Ethical and Judicial Affairs defines informed consent as follows:

> The patient's right of self-decision can be effectively exercised only if the patient possesses enough information to enable an intelligent choice. The patient should make his or her own determination on treatment. The physician's obligation is to present the medical facts accurately to the patient or to the individual responsible for the patient's care and to make recommendations for management in accordance with good medical practice. The physician has an ethical obligation to help the patient make choices from among the therapeutic alternatives consistent with good medical practice.[5]

Did you notice the word "alternatives" in the AMA's definition? Being informed means being told about all reasonable remedies, including proven effective natural therapies.

SAFETY FIRST

Nearly 50 percent of Americans use alternative medicine. Some doctors are coming around to its validity, but not enough. What are they waiting for?

In a 2003 report, Mayo Clinic doctors described the successful use of niacin to treat a woman's chronic severe migraines, which were unresponsive to prescription drugs. The doctors noted how few advances there had been in migraine prevention, adding, "Any treatment that shows efficacy for the prevention of migraine and can advance our knowledge and therapeutic options is noteworthy."[6] They were referring to the niacin, which remains ignored by mainstream medicine. It is truly unfortunate for patients when doctors are not interested in proven effective natural methods. Thankfully, you do not need permission to try the remedies presented in this book.

Migraine headaches are very painful and difficult to treat. They impair your ability to function and can be disabling. The side effects of mainstream migraine drugs, however, can also be a major problem. The purpose of this book is to provide you and the millions of other migraine sufferers with natural treatment options that have been proven safe and effective. If one of these natural remedies works for you, please tell your family, your friends, and your doctor. Hopefully, your physician will take your story to heart and pass the information on to other migraine patients who might benefit from it.

REFERENCES

Introduction

1. Wickersham, R., ed. *Drug Facts and Comparisons*. St. Louis, MO: Wolters Kluwer Health, 2009.

2. Sackett, D.L., Rosenberg W.M., Gray J.A., et al. "Evidence-based medicine: What it is and what it isn't." *BMJ* (1996); 312(7023):71–72.

3. Sackett D.L., Straus S.E., Richardson W.S., et al. *Evidence-Based Medicine: How to Practice and Teach EBM*. Edinburgh: Churchill Livingstone, 2000.

4. Than, M., Bidwell, S., Davison, C., et al. "Evidence-based emergency medicine at the 'coal face.'" *Emergency Medicine Australasia* (2005); 17(4):330–340.

5. Miller, F.G., and Rosenstein, D.L. "The therapeutic orientation to clinical trials." *New England Journal of Medicine* (2003); 384:1383–1386.

6. Dodick, D.W., and Silberstein, S.D. "Migraine prevention." *Practical Neurology* (2007); 7(6):383–393.

7. Linde, K., Allais, G., Brinkhaus, B., et al. "Acupuncture for migraine prophylaxis." *Cochrane Database Systematic Review* (2009); 21(1):CD001218.

8. Landy, S. "Migraine throughout the life cycle: treatment through the ages." *Neurology* (2004); 62(5 Suppl 2):S2–S8.

9. Evans, R.W., and Taylor, F.R. "'Natural' or alternative medications for migraine prevention." *Headache* (2006); 46(6):1012–1018.

1. What Are Migraines?

1. Penzien, D.B., Rains J.C., and Andrasik, F. "Behavioral management of recurrent headache: three decades of experience and empiricism." *Applied Psychophysiology and Biofeedback* (2002); 27(2):163–181.

2. Sun-Edelstein, C., and Mauskop, A. "Foods and supplements in the management of migraine headaches." *Clinical Journal of Pain* (2009); 25(5):446–452.

3. Landy, S. "Migraine throughout the life cycle: treatment through the ages." *Neurology* (2004); 62(5 Suppl 2):S2–S8.

4. Sacks, O. *Migraine*. Los Angeles: University of California Press, 1992.

5. Goadsby, P.J., Lipton, R.B., and Ferrari, M.D. "Migraine—Current Understanding and Treatment." *New England Journal of Medicine* (2002); 346(4):257–270.

2. Bioidentical Remedies

1. "Riboflavin Monograph." *Natural Standard: The Authority on Integrative Medicine*. 2010. www.naturalstandard.com.

2. "Riboflavin." *Mayo Clinic*. Aug. 6, 2010. www.mayoclinic.com.

3. Allee, M.R., and Baker, M.Z. "Riboflavin Deficiency." *WebMD, EMedicine*. Aug. 6, 2000. www.emedicine.medscape.com.

4. "Vitamin B2 (Riboflavin)." *University of Maryland Medical Center*. Aug. 6, 2010. www.umm.edu.

5. "Riboflavin." *Medline Plus, Trusted Health Information for You. Natural Institutes of Health*. Aug. 6, 2010. www.nlm.nih.gov/medlineplus/ency/article/002411.htm.

6. Smith, C.B. "Riboflavin in migraine." *Canadian Medical Journal* (1946); 54(6):589–591.

7. Schoenen, J., Lenaerts, M., and Bastings, E. "High-dose riboflavin as a prophylactic treatment of migraine: results of an open pilot study." *Cephalalgia* (1994); 14(5):328–329.

8. Schoenen, J., Jacquy, J., and Lenaerts, M. "Effectiveness of high-dose riboflavin in migraine prophylaxis: a randomized controlled trial." *Neurology* (1998); 50(2):466–470.

9. Boehnke, C., Reuter, U., et al. "High-dose riboflavin treatment is efficacious in migraine prophylaxis: an open study in a tertiary care centre." *European Journal of Neurology* (2004); 11(7):475–477.

10. Diener, H.C., Hartung, E., Chrubasik J., et al. "A comparative study of oral acetylsalicylic acid and metoprolol for the prophylactic treatment of migraine." *Cephalalgia* (2001); 21(2):120–128.

11. Condò, M., Posar, A., Arbizzani, A., and Parmeggiani, A. "Riboflavin prophylaxis in pediatric and adolescent migraine." *Journal of Headache and Pain* (2009); 10(5):361–365.

12. Landy, S. "Migraine throughout the life cycle: treatment through the ages." *Neurology* (2004); 62(5 Suppl 2):S2–S8.

13. Rapoport, A.M., and Bigal, M.E. "Migraine preventive therapy: current and emerging treatment options." *Neurological Science* (2005); 26(Suppl 2):S111–S120.

14. *The People's Pharmacy*. April 21, 2008. www.peoplespharmacy .com/2008/04/21/vitamin-vanquis/

15. *The People's Pharmacy*. March 16, 2009. www.peoplespharmacy .com/2009/03/16/vitamin-averts/

16. Sun-Edelstein, C., and Mauskop, A. "Alternative headache treatments: nutriceuticals, behavioral and physical treatments." *Headache* (2011); 51(3):469–483.

17. Rozen, T.D., Oshinsky, M.L., and Gebeline, C.A., et al. "Open label trial of coenzyme Q_{10} as a migraine preventive." *Cephalalgia* (2002); 22(2):137–141.

18. Sandor, S., Di Clemente, L., Coppola, G., et al. "Efficacy of coenzyme Q_{10} in migraine prophylaxis: a randomized controlled trial." *Neurology* (2005); 64(4):713–715.

19. Hershey, A.D., Powers, S.W., Vockell, A.L., et al. "Coenzyme Q_{10} deficiency and response to supplementation in pediatric and adolescent migraine." *Headache* (2007); 47(1):73–80.

20. Pines, N., and Kieff, M.B. "Magnesium sulfate in the treatment of angiospasm." *Lancet* (1933); 221(5716):577–579.

21. Mauskop, A., Altura, B.T., Cracco, R.Q., and Altura, B.M. "Intravenous magnesium sulphate relieves migraine attacks in patients with low serum ionized magnesium levels: a pilot study." *Clinical Science* (1995); 89(6):633–636.

22. Demirkaya, S., Vural, O., Dora, B., and Topcuolu, M.A. "Efficacy of intravenous magnesium sulfate in the treatment of acute migraine attacks." *Headache* (2001); 41(2):171–177.

23. Bigal, M.E., Bordini, C.A., Tepper, S.J., and Speciali, J.G. "Intravenous magnesium sulphate in the acute treatment of migraine without aura and migraine with aura. A randomized, double-blind, placebo-controlled study." *Cephalalgia* (2002); 22(5):345–353.

24. Peikert, A., Wilimzig, C., and Köhne-Volland, R. "Prophylaxis of migraine with oral magnesium: results from a prospective, multi-center, placebo-controlled and double-blind randomized study." *Cephalalgia* (1996); 16(4):257–263.

25. Pfaffenrath, V., Wessely, P., and Meyer, C. "Magnesium in the prophylaxis of migraine—a double-blind placebo-controlled study." *Cephalalgia* (1996); 16(6):436–440.

26. Köseoglu, E., Talaslioglu, A., Gönül, A.S., and Kula, M. "The effects of magnesium prophylaxis in migraine without aura." *Magnesium Research* (2008); 21(2):101–108.

27. Bryan, L. *The People's Pharmacy.* Apr 4, 2011. www.peoplespharmacy.com. Accessed June 15, 2011.

28. Peres, M.F., Zukerman, E., da Cunha Tanuri, F., et al. "Melatonin, 3 mg, is effective for migraine prevention." *Neurology* (2004); 63(4):757.

29. Murialdo, G., Fonzi, S., Costelli, P., et al. "Urinary melatonin excretion throughout the ovarian cycle in menstrually related migraine." *Cephalalgia* (1994); 14(3):205–209.

30. Peres, M.F., Masruha M.R., Zukerman E., et al. "Potential therapeutic use of melatonin in migraine and other headache disorders." *Expert Opin Investig Drugs* (2006); 15(4):367–375.

31. Peres, M.F., Zukerman, E., da Cunha Tanuri, F., et al. "Melatonin, 3 mg, is effective for migraine prevention." *Neurology* (2004); 63(4):757.

32. Miano, S., Parisi, P., Pelliccia, A., et al. "Melatonin to prevent migraine or tension-type headache in children." *Neurological Sciences* (2008); 29(4):285–287.

33. Toglia, J.U. "Is migraine due to a deficiency of pineal melatonin?" *Italian Journal of Neurological Sciences* (1986); 7(3):319–323.

34. Peres, M.F., Zukerman, E., da Cunha Tanuri, F., et al. "Melatonin, 3 mg, is effective for migraine prevention." *Neurology* (2004); 63(4):757.

35. Miano, S., Parisi, P., Pelliccia, A., et al. "Melatonin to prevent migraine or tension-type headache in children." *Neurological Sciences* (2008); 29(4):285–287.

36. Sicuteri, F. "The ingestion of serotonin precursors (L-5-hydroxytryptophan and L-tryptophan) improves migraine headache." *Headache* (1973); 13(1):19–22.

37. Boiardi, A., Crenna, P., Merati, B., et al. "5-OH-Tryptophane in migraine: clinical and neurophysiological considerations." *Journal of Neurology* (1981); 225(1):41–46.

38. Bono, G., Micieli, G., Sances, G., et al. "L-5HTP treatment in pri-

mary headaches: an attempt at clinical identification of responsive patients." *Cephalalgia* (1984); 4(3):159–165.

39. De Benedittis, G., and Massei, R. "Serotonin precursors in chronic primary headache. A double-blind cross- over study with L-5-hydroxytryptophan vs. placebo." *Journal of Neurosurgical Sciences* (1985); 29(3):239–248.

40. Titus, F., Davalos, A., Alom, J., and Codina, A. "5-Hydroxytryptophan versus methysergide in the prophylaxis of migraine." *European Neurology* (1986); 25(5):327–329.

41. Maissen C.P., and Ludin, H.P. "Comparison of the effect of 5-hydroxytryptophan and propranolol in the interval treatment of migraine." *Schweiz Med Wochenschr* (1991); 121(43):1585–1590. Abstract.

42. Grenfell, R.F. "Treatment of migraine with nicotinic acid." *American Practitioner* (1949); 3(9):542–544.

43. Atkinson, M. "Migraine headache: some clinical observations on the vascular mechanism and its control." *Annals of Internal Medicine* (1944); 21(6):990–997.

44. Velling, D.A., Dodick, D.W., and Muir, J.J. "Sustained-release niacin for prevention of migraine headache." *Mayo Clinic Proceedings* (2003); 78(6):770–771.

45. Thys-Jacobs, S. "Alleviation of migraines with therapeutic vitamin D and calcium." *Headache* (1994); 34(10):590–592.

46. Thys-Jacobs, S. "Vitamin D and calcium in menstrual migraine." *Headache* (1994); 34(9):544–546.

47. Wheeler, S.D. "Vitamin D deficiency in chronic migraine." *Headache* (2008); 48, S33(Suppl 1): S52–S53.

48. Prakash, S., Mehta, N.C., Dabhi, A.S., et al. "The prevalence of headache may be related with the latitude: a possible role of Vitamin D insufficiency?" *Journal of Headache Pain* (2010); 11(4):301–307.

49. Prakash, S., and Shah, N.D. "Chronic tension-type headache with vitamin D deficiency: casual or causal association?" *Headache* (2009); 49(8):1214—1222.

50. *The People's Pharmacy*. www.peoplespharmacy.com. April, 2010.

3. Herbal Remedies

1. Mittra, S., Datta, A., Singh, S., and Singh, A. "5-L-5-hydroxytrypta-mine-inhibiting property of feverfew: role of parthenolide content." *Acta Pharmacologica Sinica* (2000); 21(12):1106–1114.

2. Weber, J.J., O'Connor, M., Hyataka, K., et al. "Activity of partheno-lide at 5-HT2A receptors." *Journal of Natural Products* (1997); 60(6):651–653.

3. Johnson, E.S., Kadam, N.P., Hylands, D.M., and Hylands, P.J. "Effi-cacy of feverfew as prophylactic treatment of migraine." *British Med-ical Journal* (1985); 291(6495):569–573.

4. Murphy, J.J., Heptinstall, S., and Mitchell, J.R. "Randomised double-blind placebo-controlled trial of feverfew in migraine prevention." *Lancet* (1988); 2(8604):189–192.

5. Palevitch, D., Earon, G., Carasso, R. "Feverfew as a prophylactic treatment for migraine: a double-blind placebo-controlled study." *Phy-totherapy Research* (1997); 11:508–511.

6. Diener, H.C., Pfaffenrath, V., Schnitker, J., et al. "Efficacy and safety of 6.25 mg three-times-a-day feverfew CO_2-extract (MIG-99) in migraine prevention—a randomized, double-blind, multicentre, placebo-controlled study." *Cephalalgia* (2005); 25(11):1031–1041.

7. Pfaffenrath, V., Diener, H.C., Fischer, M., et al. "The efficacy and safety of Tanacetum parthenium (feverfew) in migraine prophylaxis—a double-blind, multicentre, randomized placebo-controlled dose-response study." *Cephalalgia* (2002); 22(7):523–532.

8. Pfaffenrath, V., Diener, H.C., Fischer, M., et al. "The efficacy and safety of Tanacetum parthenium (feverfew) in migraine prophylaxis—a double-blind, multicentre, randomized placebo-controlled dose-response study." *Cephalalgia* (2002); 22(7):523–532.

9. "Feverfew and migraines." *The People's Pharmacy.* Sept. 12, 2010. www.peoplespharmacy.com.

10. Pasero, G., and Marson, P. "A short history of anti-rheumatic ther-apy: Part 2, Aspirin." *Reumatismo* (2010); 62(2):148–156.

11. Roberts, A.J., O'Brien, M.E., and Subak-Sharpe, G. *Nutriceuticals: The Complete Encyclopedia of Supplements, Herbs, Vitamins and Healing Foods.* New York: Berkeley Publishing Group, 2001.

12. "White Willow Bark." *Viable Herbal Solutions.* Aug 22, 2010. www.viable-herbal.com.

13. Roberts, A.J., O'Brien, M.E., and Subak-Sharpe, G. *Nutriceuticals: The Complete Encyclopedia of Supplements, Herbs, Vitamins and Healing Foods.* New York: Berkeley Publishing Group, 2001.

14. "Willow Bark Monograph." *Natural Standard: The Authority on Integrative Medicine.* Aug 8, 2010. www.naturalstandard.com.

15. "Willow Bark Monograph." *Natural Standard: The Authority on Integrative Medicine.* Aug 8, 2010. www.naturalstandard.com.

16. Shrivastava, R., Pechadre, J.C., and John, G.W. "Tanacetum parthenium and Salix alba combination in migraine prophylaxis." *Clinical Drug Investigation* (2006); 26(5):287–296.

17. Grossman, W., and Schmidramsl, H. "An extract of Petasites hybridus is effective in the prophylaxis of migraine." *International Journal of Clinical Pharmacology and Therapeutics* (2000); 38(9):430–435.

18. Diener, H.C., Rahlfs, V.W., and Danesch, U. "The first placebo-controlled trial of a special butterbur root extract for the prevention of migraine: reanalysis of efficacy criteria." *European Neurology* (2004); 51(2):89–97.

19. Lipton, R.B., Göbel, H., Einhäupl, K.M., et al. "Petasites hybridus root (butterbur) is an effective preventive treatment for migraine." *Neurology* (2004); 63(12):2240–2244.

20. Pothmann, R., and Danesch, U. "Migraine prevention in children and adolescents: results of an open study with a special butterbur root extract." *Headache* (2005); 45(3):196–203.

21. Mustafa, T., and Srivastava, K.C. "Ginger (Zingiber officinale) in migraine headache." *Journal Ethnopharmacology* (1990); 29(3):267–273.

22. Testimonial. "GelStat for migraine headaches." November 28, 2010. GelStat Corporation. www.gelstatmigraine.com.

23. Graedon, J., and Graedon, T. "Ginger for migraines." *The People's Pharmacy.* 2008. www.peoplespharmacy.com/2008/12/06/ginger-against/

24. D'Andrea, G., Bussone, G., Allais, G., et al. "Efficacy of Ginkgolide B in the prophylaxis of migraine with aura." *Neurological Sciences* (2009); 30(Suppl 1):S121–S124.

25. Usai, S., Grazzi, L., Andrasik, F., and Bussone, G. "An innovative approach for migraine prevention in young age: a preliminary study." *Neurol Sci* (2010); 31(Suppl 1):S181–S183.

26. Esposito, M., and Carotenuto, M. "Ginkgolide B complex efficacy for brief prophylaxis of migraine in school-aged children: an open-label study." *Neurological Sciences* (2011); 32(1):79–81.

27. Wagner, W., and Nootbaar-Wagner, U. "Prophylactic treatment of migraine with gamma-linolenic and alpha-linolenic acids." *Cephalalgia* (1997); 17(2):127–130.

4. Mind and Body Remedies

1. Sargent, J.D., Walters, E.D., and Green, E.D. "The use of autogenic feedback training in a pilot study of migraine and tension headaches." *Headache* (1972); 12(3):120–124.

2. Kaushik, R., Kaushik, R.M., Mahajan, S.K., and Rajesh, V. "Biofeedback assisted diaphragmatic breathing and systematic relaxation versus propranolol in long term prophylaxis of migraine." *Complimentary Therapies in Medicine* (2005); 13(3):165–174.

3. Stokes, D.A., and Lappin, M.S. "Neurofeedback and biofeedback with 37 migraineurs: a clinical outcome study." *Behavioral and Brain Functions* (2010); 2(6):9.

4. Nestoriuc, Y., and Martin, A. "Efficacy of biofeedback for migraine: a meta-analysis." *Pain* (2007); 128(1-2):111–127.

5. RS. *The People's Pharmacy.* Dec 22, 2010. www.peoplespharmacy .com. Accessed June 15, 2011.

6. Pingping, Z. "47 cases of migraine treatment with acupuncture." *Journal of Traditional Chinese Medicine* (1992); 12(2):108–109.

7. Hesse, J., Migelvang, B., and Simonsen, H. "Acupuncture versus metoprolol in migraine prophylaxis: a randomized trial of trigger point inactivation." *Journal of Internal Medicine.* (1994); 235(5): 451–456.

8. Diener, H.C., Kronfeld, K., Boewing, G., et al. "Efficacy of acupuncture for the prophylaxis of migraine: a multicentre randomised controlled clinical trial." *Lancet Neurology* (2006); 5(4):310–316.

9. Streng, A., Linde, K., Hoppe, A., et al. "Effectiveness and tolerability of acupuncture compared with metoprolol in migraine prophylaxis." *Headache* (2006); 46(10):1492–1502.

10. Linde, K., Allais, G., Brinkhaus, B., et al. "Acupuncture for migraine prophylaxis." *Cochrane Database Systematic Review* (2009); 21(1):CD001218.

5. Preventing Migraines in Children and Adolescents

1. Longo, G., Rudoi, I., Iannuccelli, M., et al. "Treatment of essential headache in developmental age with L-5-HTP (cross over double-blind study versus placebo)." La Pediatria medica e chirurgica: Medical and Surgical Pediatrics (1984); 6(2):241–245.

2. De Giorgis, G., Miletto, R., Iannuccelli, M., et al. "Headache in association with sleep disorders in children: a psychodiagnostic evaluation and controlled clinical study—L-5-HTP versus placebo." *Drugs under Experimental and Clinical Research* (1987); 13(7):425–433.

3. Pothmann, R., Danesch, U. "Migraine prevention in children and adolescents: results of an open study with a special butterbur root extract." *Headache* (2005); 45(3):196–203.

4. Hershey, A.D., Powers, S.W., Vockell, A.L., et al. "Coenzyme Q_{10} deficiency and response to supplementation in pediatric and adolescent migraine." *Headache* (2007); 47(1):73–80.

5. Miano, S., Parisi, P., Pelliccia, A., et al. "Melatonin to prevent migraine or tension-type headache in children." *Neurological Sciences* (2008); 29(4):285–287.

6. Condò, M., Posar, A., Arbizzani, A., Parmeggiani, A. "Riboflavin prophylaxis in pediatric and adolescent migraine." *Journal of Headache and Pain* (2009); 10(5):361–365.

7. Usai, S., Grazzi, L., Andrasik, F., and Bussone, G. "An innovative approach for migraine prevention in young age: a preliminary study." *Neurol Sci* (2010); 31(Suppl 1):S181–S183.

8. Esposito, M., and Carotenuto, M. "Ginkgolide B complex efficacy for brief prophylaxis of migraine in school-aged children: an open-label study." *Neurological Sciences* (2011); 32(1):79–81.

6. Natural Remedies for Acute Migraines

1. Pines, N., and Kieff, M.B. "Magnesium sulfate in the treatment of angiospasm." *Lancet* (1933); 221(5716):577–579.

2. Mauskop, A., Altura, B.T., Cracco, R.Q., and Altura, B.M. "Intra-

venous magnesium sulphate relieves migraine attacks in patients with low serum ionized magnesium levels: a pilot study." *Clinical Science* (1995); 89(6):633–636.

3. Demirkaya, S., Vural, O., Dora, B., Topcuolu, M.A. "Efficacy of intravenous magnesium sulfate in the treatment of acute migraine attacks." *Headache* (2001); 41(2):171-177.

4. Bigal, M.E., Bordini, C.A., Tepper S.J., and Speciali J.G. "Intravenous magnesium sulphate in the acute treatment of migraine without aura and migraine with aura. A randomized, double-blind, placebo-controlled study." *Cephalalgia* (2002); 22(5):345–353.

5. Atkinson, M. "Migraine headache: some clinical observations on the vascular mechanism and its control." *Annals of Internal Medicine* (1944), 21(6):990–997.

6. Grenfell, R.F. "Treatment of migraine with nicotinic acid." *American Practitioner* (1949); 3(9):542–544.

7. Hall, J.A. "Enhancing niacin's effect for migraine." *Cortlandt Forum* (1991); 46:47

8. Prousky, J., and Seely, D. "The treatment of migraines and tension-type headaches with intravenous and oral niacin (nicotinic acid): systematic review of the literature." *Nutrition Journal* (2005); 4:3.

9. Gedye, A. "Hypothesized treatment for migraines using low doses of tryptophan, niacin, calcium, caffeine and acetylsalicylic acid." *Medical Hypotheses* (2001); 56(1):91–94.

10. Prousky, J., and Sykes, E. "Two case reports on the treatment of acute migraine with niacin. Its hypothetical mechanism of action upon calcitonin-gene related peptide and platelets." *Journal of Orthomolecular Medicine* (2003); 18(2):108–110.

11. Smith, C.B. "Riboflavin in migraine." *Canadian Medical Journal* (1946); 54(6):589–591.

12. Thys-Jacobs, S. "Vitamin D and calcium in menstrual migraine." *Headache* (1994); 34(9):544–546.

13. Cady, R.K., Schreiber, C.P., Beach, M.E., et al. "GelStat Migraine (sublingually administered feverfew and ginger compound) for acute treatment of migraine when administered during the mild pain phase." *Medical Science Monitor* (2005); 11(9):P165–P169.

14. Melchart, D., Thormaehlen, J., Hager, S., et al. "Acupuncture versus

placebo versus sumatriptan for early treatment of migraine headaches: a randomized controlled trial." *Journal of Internal Medicine* (2003); 253(2):181–188.

15. Li, Y., Liang, F., Yang, X., et al. "Acupuncture for treating acute attacks of migraine: a randomized controlled trial." *Headache* (2009); 49(6):805–816.

Conclusion

1. Silberstein, S.D., Neto, W., Schmitt, J., and Jacobs, D. "Topiramate in migraine prevention: results of a large controlled trial." *Archives of Neurology* (2004); 61(4):490–495.

2. Johnson, E.S., Kadam, N.P., Hylands, D.M., and Hylands, P.J. "Efficacy of feverfew as prophylactic treatment of migraine." *British Medical Journal* (1985); 291(6495):569–573.

3. Peres, M.F., Zukerman, E., da Cunha Tanuri, F., et al. "Melatonin, 3 mg, is effective for migraine prevention." *Neurology* (2004); 63(4):757.

4. Pothmann, R., Danesch, U. "Migraine prevention in children and adolescents: results of an open study with a special butterbur root extract." *Headache* (2005); 45(3):196–203.

5. American Medical Association Council on Ethical and Judicial Affairs. *Code of Medical Ethics, 1998–1999 Edition.* Chicago, IL: American Medical Association.

6. Velling, D.A., Dodick, D.W., and Muir, J.J. "Sustained-release niacin for prevention of migraine headache." *Mayo Clinic Proceedings* (2003); 78(6):770–771.

ABOUT THE AUTHOR

Jay S. Cohen, MD, is an Adjunct (Voluntary) Associate Professor of Family and Preventive Medicine and of Psychiatry at the University of California, San Diego. He has published numerous scientific papers in leading medical journals and has written articles for *Newsweek*, *Life Extension Magazine*, and *Bottom Line Health*. He is the author of a number of books on natural therapies for common medical conditions, including *Over Dose: The Case Against the Drug Companies*.

Dr. Cohen has spoken extensively on how to avoid medication side effects and when to use natural remedies instead of prescription drugs. He has been a keynote speaker at major medical conferences and has debated drug safety with top officials at the US Food and Drug Administration.

Dr. Cohen splits his time between his psychiatry and psychopharmacology practice in Del Mar, CA, and his research and writing. Originally from Philadelphia, where he attended Temple Medical School, he has lived in Del Mar for thirty-five years.

INDEX

Acupuncture, 101–105,
    127–129, 132
Auras, 14, 17–18, 40,
    120–121

Biofeedback, 93–101, 132
Butterbur, 78–83, 109–111,
    132

Calciferol. *See* Vitamin D.
Coenzyme Q$_{10}$, 30–35, 111,
    132
CoQ$_{10}$. *See* Coenzyme Q$_{10}$.

Feverfew, 67–74, 130, 132
5-HTP. *See* 5-
    Hydroxytryptophan.
5-Hydroxytryptophan,
    46–53, 108–109, 132

Gamma linolenic acid,
    89–92
GelStat, 85–86, 126–127
Ginger, 83–86, 126–127
Ginkgo biloba, 87–89, 114–115
GLA. *See* Gamma linolenic
    acid.

Imitrex. *See* Sumatriptan.

Magnesium, 35–43, 118–121,
    132
Maxalt. *See* Rizatriptan.
Melatonin, 43–46, 112–113,
    132
Metoprolol, 103–105
Migraines
    acute, 117–129
    causes of, 17
    in children and
        adolescents, 107–116
    definition of, 14–15
    remedies for, *See* Remedies.
    symptoms of, 14–15
    triggers of, 18

Niacin, 53–59, 121–125
    flush, 54, 58–59, 122–125
Nicotinic acid. *See* Niacin.

Pellagra, 53
Propranolol, 52, 96–98

Remedies
    for acute migraines,
        117–129
    bioidentical, 21–65
    in combination, 133
    herbal, 67–92

for migraines in children
    and adolescents,
    107–116
mind and body, 93–106
Riboflavin, 21–30, 113–114,
    125, 132
Rizatriptan, 117

Salacin, 74
Sumatriptan, 117

Topiramate, 130–131
Topamax. *See* Topiramate.

Ubiquinone. *See*
    Coenzyme Q$_{10}$.

Vitamin B$_2$. *See* Riboflavin.
Vitamin B$_3$. *See* Niacin.
Vitamin D, 59–65,
    125–126

White Willow, 74–78, 132

Zolmitriptan, 117
Zomig. *See*
    Zolmitriptan.

OTHER SQUAREONE TITLES OF INTEREST

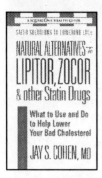

NATURAL ALTERNATIVES TO LIPITOR, ZOCOR, & OTHER STATIN DRUGS

What to Use and Do to Help Lower Your Bad Cholesterol

Jay S. Cohen, MD

Elevated cholesterol and C-reactive proteins are markers linked to heart attack, stroke, and other cardiovascular disorders. While modern science has created a group of drugs known as statins to combat these problems, nearly 50 percent of the people who take them experience side effects. This guide explains the problems caused by statins and highlights the most effective natural alternatives.

$7.95 • 144 pages • 4 x 7-inch mass paperback • ISBN 978-0-7570-0286-1

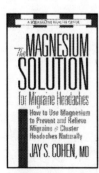

THE MAGNESIUM SOLUTION FOR MIGRAINE HEADACHES

How to Use Magnesium to Prevent and Relieve Migraine & Cluster Headaches Naturally

Jay S. Cohen, MD

More than 30 million people in North America suffer from migraine headaches. While a number of drugs are used to treat migraines, they come with a risk of side effects. But there is a safe alternative—magnesium. This guide shows how magnesium can treat migraines, and pinpoints the best magnesium to use and the proper dosage.

$5.95 • 96 pages • 4 x 7-inch mass paperback • ISBN 978-0-7570-0256-4

WHAT YOU MUST KNOW ABOUT VITAMINS, MINERALS, HERBS & MORE

Choosing the Nutrients That Are Right for You

Pamela Wartian Smith, MD, MPH

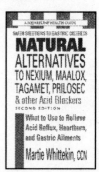

What You Must Know About Vitamins, Minerals, Herbs & More guides you in restoring and maintaining health through the wise use of nutrients. Part One discusses the individual nutrients necessary for well-being, Part Two offers nutritional programs for a wide variety of health concerns, and Part Three presents supplementation plans. Whether you want to preserve good health or overcome a medical condition, this book will give you the information you need to make the best nutritional choices possible.

$15.95 • 448 pages • 6 x 9-inch quality paperback • ISBN 978-0-7570-0233-5

NATURAL ALTERNATIVES TO NEXIUM, MAALOX, TAGAMET, PRILOSEC & OTHER ACID BLOCKERS

What to Use to Help Relieve Acid Reflex, Heartburn, and Gastric Ailments

Martie Whittekin, CCN

Natural Alternatives to Nexium examines the underlying causes of acid-related gastric ailments. Most important, it highlights effective natural alternatives—both those that provide immediate relief and those that offer long-term relief. If you suffer from the pain of recurrent gastric upset, this book can make a profound difference in the quality of your life.

$7.95 • 272 pages • 4 x 7-inch mass paperback • ISBN 978-0-7570-0210-6

For more information about our books, visit our website at
www.squareonepublishers.com